WORLD TRENDS IN MEDICAL EDUCATION

THE MACY FOUNDATION SERIES ON INTERNATIONAL PROBLEMS OF MEDICAL EDUCATION

EDITED BY ELIZABETH PURCELL

WORLD TRENDS IN MEDICAL EDUCATION

Faculty, Students, and Curriculum

Report of A Macy Conference

Published for the JOSIAH MACY, JR. FOUNDATION
by THE JOHNS HOPKINS PRESS, Baltimore and London

The Johns Hopkins Press, Baltimore, Maryland 21218
The Johns Hopkins Press Ltd., London

Library of Congress Catalog Card Number 79–144335

International Standard Book Number 0–8018–1270–4

CONTENTS

INTRODUCTION

The past two decades have been characterized by an unparalleled ferment in medical education throughout the world. In an effort to document and analyze these changes, the Josiah Macy, Jr. Foundation convened an international conference in September 1969, the proceedings of which are reported in this volume. Since a previous Macy conference had been focused primarily on the developing countries, as reported in *Medical Schools for the Modern World,** a principal emphasis in this conference was on European countries. The representatives of two countries, Japan and India, were not able to attend but they prepared papers that are included in this book.

The open admissions policies pose severe problems in a number of countries. The French are responding to this issue by establishing a two-year basic science curriculum, after which students are "sorted out" for careers in medicine, dentistry, nursing, related health professions, or technology.

A precipitous expansion in the number of schools, as has occurred recently in India and Brazil, and earlier in the Philippines, presents the dilemma of quantity versus quality in the graduates and of an adequate qualified faculty.

In Japan and in several European countries, rigid control of the medical curriculum by a national ministry of education poses a major obstacle in efforts to reform medical education.

The percentage of women studying medicine has soared in Western Europe. A major problem, however, is their lack of dedication to the practice of medicine. In Great Britain, 75 per cent do no medical work after graduation. In the Communist countries of Eastern Europe there are governmental programs for the maximum effective utilization of the services of women graduates. The organization of the health services allows them to work on a nine-to-five basis and the financial benefit is an important factor when the income of a husband is low.

Relationships with medical students was a problem foremost in the minds of all the participants and dominated the discussions. The demands of the students for open admissions, for curriculum reform, for the abolition of grading systems, and for a dominant voice in determining university policy, were recurring themes.

These are just a few of the trends that were the substance of the conference.

* Edited by John Z. Bowers (Baltimore: The Johns Hopkins Press for the Josiah Macy, Jr. Foundation, 1970).

The Macy Foundation wishes once again to express its appreciation to The Rockefeller Foundation for the opportunity to convene the conference at the lovely Villa Serbelloni in Bellagio, Lake Como, Italy. Sixteen countries join in a global "thank you" to Charlotte and John Marshall not only for their hospitality but for the intellectual elegance that they brought to our conference.

JOHN Z. BOWERS, M.D.
President
Josiah Macy, Jr. Foundation

WORLD TRENDS IN MEDICAL EDUCATION

BENJAMIN VIEL V.
Professor of Hygiene and Preventive and Social Medicine
University of Chile
Faculty of Medicine
Santiago, Chile

SPANISH-SPEAKING LATIN AMERICA

THE COLONIZATION of part of Latin America by Spain began during the reign of the Catholic King Ferdinand V, known in history for his support of Columbus's travels across the Atlantic. He is not so favorably remembered for the expulsion of the Jews and Arabs and the establishment of the Inquisition, that horrible institution that existed for more than 300 years.

The expulsion of the Arabs, regarded as a necessary step for the unification of Spain, brought as a consequence a severe and regrettable diminution of specialized manpower; it took more than a century to recover from the loss of the craftsmen who were forced to leave.

The expulsion of the Jews was an even harder blow because with them left a great number of scientists who had been principally responsible for the fine scientific tradition of medieval Spain.

The Inquisition was founded to keep Spain united under one ruler and to ensure that the population would have only one religion—the Catholic faith. But the cultural atmosphere of Spain began to smell of burning human flesh; freedom of thought was abolished and natural sciences became a very dangerous topic of discussion. Since the conclusions obtained from direct observation of nature do not always agree with the Bible, students of nature were in constant danger of being accused of witchcraft.

No wonder then that the study of medicine was not an attractive pursuit. Since medicine must be based on natural sciences, those who intended to practice it were in continual danger of being regarded with distrust, unless they restricted themselves to the empirical principles accepted by their masters and taught to them in universities that were

---

Benjamin Viel received his M.D. from the University of Chile in 1938, the M.P.H. from the Harvard School of Public Health in 1940, and the D.P.H. from the Johns Hopkins School of Public Health in 1944. Since 1947 he has been professor of preventive medicine at the medical school of the University of Chile. He was director of the university medical school from 1952 to 1963. He has been a WHO consultant and a visiting professor at several universities on the American continent.

closely observed by the Inquisition leaders and where any kind of research was considered suspicious.

History of Higher Education

This was the atmosphere exported to the Americas. In its dominions Spain founded several universities, all of them under the same repressive spirit that existed in the motherland.

In 1713 the municipal government of Santiago, Colony of Chile, requested from the King the necessary support to found a university. Permission was granted and a university was founded to teach theology, law, philosophy, mathematics, and medicine. The latter two subjects attracted no students. Most of the few physicians who practiced in Chile before independence were Europeans whose degrees had been revalidated by the University of San Marcos in Peru.

After independence, in 1818, the traditional scholastic universities were closed. The recently born countries looked to France as a source of inspiration for their philosophy—the ideals of the French Revolution and of Napoleon were the inspiration of the intellectuals of that era. The young republics of Latin America copied the Napoleonic Code for the administration of their laws and for their systems of education. Primary school was available to all, secondary school to those who intended to pursue an intellectual career, and, finally, the university to those who intended to follow a liberal profession such as law, medicine, engineering, pharmacy, and so forth.

Each new country founded a university, all of them governed by the same general principles. The university consisted of a group of professional schools united under a central administration but with no other relationship to each other. In those countries where there was no scientific cultural tradition the professional schools had almost no research facilities.

These universities were well suited to the kind of society that existed in Latin America during the nineteenth century. Middle-class fathers wanted to send their sons to study liberal professions that would allow them to earn their livings and to eventually become wealthy. This in turn would allow them to improve their social status and associate with the landowner group that held political and economic power.

The professional schools were so independent that in not a single case were they united in a university campus. Medical schools were located far away from engineering schools, as if medicine and biology had no relationship to mathematics. Schools of pharmacy, the only place where it was possible to study chemistry as a principal subject, had departments of biology separate from the medical schools and teachers colleges.

Society wanted the university as a place where it was possible to study a liberal profession, not as a center for the advancement of knowledge. Students regarded the university as a means of obtaining a degree, not as a place where they could study to become scientists.

If we look at Latin American medical schools of that time we see a group of highly qualified, prestigious physicians teaching students the principles of medical practice instead of giving them an approach to scientific methods that would allow the students to think for themselves. The medieval scholastic university was dead but teaching was still more empirical than scientific.

If the objective of the medical school was to train practitioners, nothing could have been better than to select professors from among the most successful practitioners of the community. Since the universities were unable to pay satisfactory salaries the professors worked part-time; they came to the university only to lecture and very seldom to give practical demonstrations to the students.

The professors of anatomy, almost the only subject in which the students could learn by using their hands, were surgeons who taught anatomy as a basic tool in order to perform surgery; structure was in no way related to function. When a chair of surgery became vacant it was almost always filled by a professor of anatomy.

The professors of physiology, also practicing clinicians, had no connection with the surgeons. Since they were so short of experimental and demonstration materials, most of the teaching was done by lecture with chalk and blackboard. It was not at all unusual for a professor of physiology to become a professor of clinical medicine.

Biochemistry was chiefly taught by the most able and prestigious owner of a clinical laboratory and the knowledge acquired there was much more closely related to blood analysis than to the metabolic processes of the human being.

The subjects presented to the students were so badly co-ordinated that it was not unusual for different professors to defend contradictory opinions. It was also not unusual for students to receive, for example, several lectures on vitamins in the physiology course and in the biochemistry course, or to study leukemia in clinical medicine as well as in pediatrics. Examples of this time-consuming and repetitive system of describing the same disease at different stages of a student's medical education could be multiplied.

Graduates came out of medical school with a great deal of theoretical knowledge, very little practical ability, and almost no scientific method. Feeling insecure, they spent their mornings as volunteers in charity hospitals and the remainder of the day waiting for private patients who would increase in number to the point where they would produce an income.

The non-paying charity patients were human guinea pigs on whom the young doctors practiced in order to acquire the minimal ability to practice medicine, an ability they should have acquired in medical school.

Medicine in the Twentieth Century

At the beginning of this century things began to change. Latin American professors of medicine and surgery visited European universities and, using Germany, England, and France as models, began placing greater emphasis on the basic sciences, taught by specialists and not by amateur clinicians as in the past. Some medical schools offered contracts to European scientists to come and teach biology, physiology, pharmacology, and pathology.

Some young graduates were sent abroad on fellowships, and for the first time medical faculties began to compete to finance full-time professors and assistants in basic science chairs.

In the medical school where I studied from 1931 to 1936 there was only one full-time professor, an Italian from Padua. Today that school has more than 150 full-time professors, most of them in basic sciences and preventive medicine; unfortunately very few of them are in clinics.

World War II cut Latin America off from Europe. The successful clinicians' customary visits to the continent were discontinued, and Latin America began to look more and more to North American universities. An increasing number of fellowships to United States' medical schools were offered and when those graduates returned they started the revolution in medical teaching that is still going on.

The Current Status of Medical Teaching

Almost without exception basic sciences are now taught by full-time specialists who also carry on research. All are well trained in scientific methods and aware that only those things that we do with our hands are really remembered; they try to train students in the laboratory rather than in the auditorium whenever feasible.

Since practical teaching can be given only to small groups, selection for admission to medical school was seen as the only answer. Today a great many medical schools select their students and limit the first-year class.

We are living in a transitional period, however, and the big change in basic sciences has not yet occurred in the clinics. In most of our medical schools clinical teaching is still in the hands of part-time, highly successful clinicians. Not all of them understand that it is more important to teach how to think scientifically in front of a patient than to give a lecture describing the most frequent symptoms of a particular disease.

Nor do all the clinicians have communication with the professors of basic sciences. Because of this unfortunate void the students feel that basic sciences are not related to clinical subjects, since their clinical professors have become so successful without a knowledge of them.

Curriculum

Tradition is still too strong. Only very few medical schools—among the best examples are the Universidad del Valle in Cali, Colombia, and the Universidad de Antioquia in Medellin, Colombia—understand that medical teaching may be compared to the erection of a tall building. Some subjects, such as biology, anatomy, physiology, psychology, and sociology, should act as supporting pillars, extending throughout the entire curriculum, while others should be considered as floors supported by the pillars, thus enabling the students to trace deviations from the normal, not as related to one particular organ or system but to the individual as a whole.

To teach such an integrated curriculum requires a close relationship between all subjects. This cannot be realized without a reasonable departmentalization in which all the members are employed full time.

We do have curriculum committees which should be responsible for the integration of the curriculum through all the years of medical school. But only the basic scientists have enough time to discuss curriculum; the clinicians finish their teaching and then go off to their private practices. When they do have an opportunity to get together for a meeting the committees' decisions are not always recognized by all of its members, and by the end of the discussion the clinicians have to leave. Co-ordination exists on paper but not in reality. These committees will begin to function only when teaching in the medical schools becomes a full-time occupation.

The Chair System

Most of our schools still maintain a system of independent chairs so isolated that sometimes they resemble feudal kingdoms; they have very little or no relationship to each other. This obsolete independent chair system is the major obstacle to integrated teaching. The number of chairs is proliferating, for the ideal of a specialist in nephrology, for example, is to become a professor and to have a chair devoted to diseases of the kidney.

One of the aims of the student revolution is to destroy the chair system and to substitute departments in which the chairs would be integrated. The main problem we are facing is the traditional attitude of professors against having departments. All of them agree in theory that it would be preferable to have a single department of medicine rather than different chairs for various subjects in medicine, but we have not yet been able to accomplish this transition.

Teaching Comprehensive Medicine

We tell our students that a man cannot be isolated; that, for example, he does not have heart disease exclusively; he is sick and his disease must be considered in total, even to the repercussions it may have in his family and social environment.

In spite of our saying this, the students observe that their professors are not co-ordinated among themselves and that the various subjects in the curriculum are not as integrated as they should be. They study medicine without knowing the fundamental concepts of biochemistry and physiology; then in another year they are frequently taught the study of pathology or psychiatry. But almost never will their professors point out to them the social implications of the cases they are studying.

Most Latin American medical schools, especially those that select their students, can now claim in all justice that they have a much more practical approach to teaching. During the clinical year the students are subjected to the clerkship system in the medical and surgical wards, and as a result they are much better prepared to practice medicine immediately after graduation than they were when they were given only theoretical lectures. On the other hand, the clinical professors are still part-time, have little communication with the full-time basic scientists, and must leave the hospital at mid-day to earn their living in private practice.

The part-time system of the clinical group is responsible for a great deal of wasted time in medical teaching, while the independent chair system is responsible for the inco-ordination with which different subjects are taught.

The unfortunate divorce of basic and clinical subjects gives the students the erroneous concept that a profound knowledge of basic sciences is important only for those who are going into research and that it is not essential for those who intend to be practitioners. This leads the students to believe that the best course is to memorize symptoms in order to make diagnoses and to memorize medicaments in order to prescribe.

Defects such as those I have described are partly responsible for the student unrest and for their criticism, but they are not the only cause of it. Medicine and medical teaching are changing, but society is changing much faster.

The old charitable hospitals of Latin America are being replaced by hospitals administered by social security agencies and patients are no longer receiving medical care as a favor or as charity but as a right.

The liberal professions, especially medicine, are more and more becoming social professions. Physicians are being employed by medical institutions in increasing numbers. No longer does the young graduate work as a volunteer in a charity hospital, acquiring the skill to become a successful practitioner with a large and profitable private practice. Unfortunately, however, a great many clinical professors have been accustomed to that way of life.

Hospital Teaching

When I was a medical student, hospital patients were extremely useful for teaching because most of them were afflicted with acute infectious diseases. The entire picture could be developed in the hospital: it would show a man being very sick and then recovering and leaving, almost ready to go back to work.

Today, with the incidence of infectious disease declining, most hospital patients have acute episodes of chronic disease and when they leave the hospital they are still quite sick. Students, therefore, are learning a type of medicine that consists primarily of observing acute episodes of chronic ailments.

Under such conditions the students are given only a very limited picture of ill health; they can never learn the proper management of chronic disease until we establish the follow-up system for teaching purposes.

The students feel very strongly that the type of medicine they are being taught is suitable only for treating the affluent group of society and that it is utterly unrelated to the present conditions or to the future society in which they are going to be practicing.

They complain that basic principles of sociology are not included in the curriculum; they want to learn more about industrial diseases, nutrition, and preventive medicine, not as separate subjects but infiltrating the entire curriculum. As practitioners they want to be able to apply scientific method and at the same time be teachers or promoters in the emerging society.

Preventive Medicine

Departments of preventive medicine are a relatively new concept in Latin America but their number is increasing. When I was a student, preventive medicine meant sanitation—water supply and sewage. Today we have a much better approach to preventive medicine, but it is in a separate chair, unrelated to clinical medicine and other subjects, so the students think of it as a different specialty, not as something that should be included in the clinical curriculum.

One good approach would be to try to make professors of medicine understand that preventive medicine is not a field one pursues at one's desk, say comparing vital statistics; it should be practiced in the community and in the home. This approach is not very common and not at all popular with professors of medicine, who think we are wasting the students' time. My criticism of the schools of public health in Latin America is that they are helping to advance the idea that preventive medicine is a specialty unrelated to clinical medicine.

We do not know exactly what the future holds but we can guess from the present trend that medical practice is going to be completely different, patterned more or less after the present British system. Thinking along these lines, the most important contribution preventive medicine could make would be in demonstration areas that have a broad approach to human ecology, where students are shown what can be done in a community when we apply scientific methods and good medical practice and when clinical and preventive medicine are combined as one subject.

We have been trying to develop this idea, and we now have a demonstration area in our department in Santiago. All my assistants are clinicians—pediatricians and obstetricians who, up until now, have been the most receptive group of clinicians in Chile to the concept of integrated medical care. In Latin American countries this combination of pediatricians and obstetricians could take care of 70 per cent of the health problems because we have a young population.

If we are able to add to this group other professionals, such as social workers, nurses, and sociologists, we will have a department that should be better qualified to deal with human ecology than preventive medicine alone. The solution to our health care problems is to have integrated demonstration areas in which we can experiment with new concepts that we hope will be widely applied in the future.

Student Unrest

The common accusation of Latin American students that the medicine they are being taught is not related to the present or future society is encouraging the students' revolutions. These are common occurrences now on the Latin American continent, and it is too early to judge what the final effect will be. In most cases I think they should be regarded as constructive, and it is hoped that the students will succeed in getting rid of the elements that would like to use the universities as tools to attain political power.

Conclusion

In my opinion, reforms in medical education in Latin America should be based on the principle that we should teach fewer facts and place a great deal more emphasis on how to think within the framework of the scientific method; that we should break out of the ivory tower and try to make the medical school relate more to the community; that we should have schools in which the teacher thinks of the university as his life and not as a part-time career that gives him more prestige in the community where he practices. Only if we attain these objectives will we be able to cope successfully with the unrest of our students.

ROBERTO F. SANTOS
Rector
Federal University of Bahia
Salvador, Bahia, Brazil

BRAZIL

Brazil occupies an area of 8.5 million square kilometers. Between the time the first census was taken in 1872 and the most recent one in 1960 the population increased from roughly 10 million to 70 million. The next census will be in 1970, when it is estimated that the population will have risen to 95 million.

Most of the population is concentrated along the coastal areas. Economically and demographically the interior near the Amazon is of little importance. The northeast, where I come from, is a problem area, with a population of about 35 million and an average per capita income of about U.S. $120 a year.

In 1872 the population density was 1.17 per square kilometer; in 1960 it was 8.34. While the density appears low it does not take into account the huge area that is relatively uninhabited and probably uninhabitable, even with today's technological knowledge. Every dollar put into that area has been wasted so far.

Health Problems

Thirty per cent of the population is under the age of nine, 42 per cent is fourteen and under, and 53 per cent is under nineteen.

The source of many of the health-related problems in Brazil is basically economic and only indirectly medical. Eighteen thousand out of every 100,000 deaths are of children under fourteen years of age; in the United States and Denmark the figure is 3,000 for that age group. There is nothing exceptional about Brazil, compared to other underdeveloped areas, in regard to causes of death in that age range.

For every 100,000 deaths, 26,000 are in the fifteen- to fifty-nine-year age group, as compared to 12,000 in Denmark and 15,000 in the United States. Deaths in this group are mainly attributable to schistosomiasis, Chaga's disease, and tuberculosis. In the sixty years and over age group, whereas in Denmark and the United States the figure exceeds 80,000 out of 100,000 deaths, in Brazil it is 56,000.

To compare two areas of Brazil, out of 100,000 deaths in the northeast, 27,000 are children under fourteen years, whereas in the affluent southeast only 10,000 deaths are in that age group. The figure is about the same in the fifteen- to fifty-nine-year range.

Higher Education

Established in 1808, the Federal University of Bahia was the first institution of higher education in Brazil, created as an isolated professional academy having no connection with the existing educational system. Subsequently, there was a proliferation of isolated institutions dedicated to training personnel for specific professions—medicine, law, engineering, economics, and so forth. Each school was complete in itself in the sense that it offered all courses required for the degree it gave, including those in the basic sciences. Until just over three decades ago, indeed, all teaching and research in mathematics, physics, chemistry, and biology was related to what a particular school considered necessary for its students' training.

In the 1930's the first true universities began operations with programs based primarily on their previous experience in professional education. For the first time, mathematics, physics, and biology were taught as independent subjects, without the limitations that had been imposed by the objectives of a particular school.

But the tradition of isolation was so strong that between the 1930's and 1960's the integration of the various schools as a university was limited to administrative matters; from the standpoint of teaching and research each unit was autonomous. Sociologically, this evolution was to be expected.

Our society felt the need for physicians before it recognized the need for mathematicians, physicists, and chemists. For many years those who controlled the country derived their incomes from traditional agricultural sources; new developments were ignored. It was considered important, however, to have good physicians to take care of the small fraction of the population that held all the power.

In our history, then, the physician did not receive his training in institutions dedicated to education or to scientific research. From the beginning, training was virtually limited to the acquisition of certain skills through an apprenticeship system. Teaching in the basic sciences was limited to transmitting information directly applicable to the practice of medicine. This was made worse by the fact that schools of medicine and engineering were almost the only institutions teaching any science. Until some thirty years ago even science teachers in secondary schools were either physicians or civil engineers—many still are.

Between 1964 and 1969 student enrollment in all universities increased from 140,000 to 278,000. In part, this was the result of a general increase in available funds, as well as the fact that in 1960 there was a change in the government's philosophy regarding the financing of education.

Until the late 1950's almost all federal funds went to higher education, with the understanding that the universities would prepare the future leaders of the country. In the 1950's funds were abundant for the relatively small number of university students, and we were able to put some of the money into better quality research and service to the community.

Secondary and primary education had not developed to the same degree because it was supported by extremely limited private, state, and municipal resources. With the shift in the government's orientation, in 1960 federal funds began to flow into secondary education. This was a sound philosophy, but it put the universities in a very difficult financial situation.

Countries that are struggling for social and economic development are apt to go into a pendulum-type of movement—to exaggerate certain factors in one direction and then go all the way in the other direction.

Medical Education

In 1900 there were only three medical schools in Brazil. Beginning in 1950, however, in spite of the pressure not to build additional schools, new medical schools were opened on an entirely unplanned basis until they have now reached the incredible total of seventy-two!

In 1951 total medical student enrollment was 9,000; in 1968 enrollment had reached 25,000. In 1967, 2,075 physicians were graduated. Brazil now has 40,000 physicians for an estimated population of 90 million—a ratio of 1:2,250.

Not long ago the educational authorities were very concerned about the quality of medical school graduates and how to improve their training. They have tried to keep the intake down but the demand has become so tremendous that this has not been possible. Quality has certainly been sacrificed for quantity. The number of medical schools is increasing and yet we are unable to prepare enough teachers to staff them.

The older medical schools are connected with universities and are located in the larger cities. The newer schools are being established in small towns that have reasonably good hospitals for teaching purposes. The hospitals must meet the requirements of a committee of experts that visits the buildings, verifies the available equipment, and investigates the backgrounds of the future staff members. The requirements are rather loose, however, and have become more so over the past few years.

Requirements for Admission

Before 1960 the older medical schools took in from 60 to 100 freshmen a year; now they take in an average of 200. The newer schools admit an average of 100 each.

Candidates must have had at least twelve years of education—five of primary and seven of secondary school—and have reached the minimum age of seventeen. There are seven or eight candidates for each opening and the entrance examination is fiercely competitive.

Curriculum

There is no premedical course, primarily because, except in the professional schools, there are very few physicists or chemists in Brazil. In their first year the students begin to study human anatomy, biochemistry, physiology, and other basic sciences.

Some medical schools have made changes in the entrance requirements, however, with the idea of offering a preprofessional basic science course. Instead of students starting with basic medical sciences they have two or three semesters in the premedical sciences. We are hoping to extend the medical curriculum to six years. In the older medical schools the development of medical education has been limited chiefly because of the lack of basic science courses.

Until the late 1950's almost all our medical schools followed the same curriculum. In the beginning of the 1960's the principle of the minimum curriculum was adopted. Today we have a basic or minimum curriculum for each of the professions that require legal certification of their graduates. The curricula are usually laid down in broad terms—the medical curriculum, for example, consists of twelve subjects and allows for considerable diversity and experimentation.

No two medical schools have identical curricula. Theoretically, the curriculum is traditional, or else one that was fashionable in the

United States when that particular school opened and was making efforts to reform its curriculum. In general, elective courses are encouraged, especially in the more developed schools.

A one-year internship was adopted by all the schools ten to twelve years ago. Residency programs were introduced recently at all major medical schools and they are proving to be fairly satisfactory. The smaller schools have no residency programs.

Training the Teachers

The preparation of teachers is a singularly important problem in a developing country. Twenty years ago the Brazilian government established an agency that specializes in providing opportunities to train teachers for higher education, including medicine. By awarding fellowships for study, both in Brazil and abroad, that agency supports the concept of "islands of excellence" in the more advanced Brazilian universities; in spite of some fluctuations, the results have been quite favorable.

In the medical schools, the vast majority of teachers, whom the students so often look upon as models, still maintain successful practices and work only part-time in the schools. Most of the schools are greatly concerned about improving teaching, but because these part-time clinicians have been away from the more advanced centers for some time it would be difficult for them to find the time to make a better adjustment to their responsibilities. Each of the schools has a few in key positions who try to upgrade their work, but this is certainly not enough.

In the older schools, inbreeding is the rule. At Bahia, for example, there are only three faculty members who are not graduates of the medical school.

The government has abolished the system that prevailed since the first medical schools were established. It consisted essentially of the following features: Lifetime tenure; strict association of a tenured professor and his specialty which, in any given school, sometimes became his personal property in the sense that no decision could be made on teaching or research in that subject without his consent; selection of professors based on a complex system of competitive examinations to assess qualities that are no longer considered of particular importance in the modern academic environment.

With the termination of this *ex cathedra* system, decisions regarding teaching and research in a given area of knowledge are now made by a vote of all members of a department. We cannot as yet determine the long-range effectiveness of this system, although we have observed some fruitful results in only a few months.

One very clearcut problem in Brazil is that we are apt to overdevelop certain services and overlook others. What is worse, there is a tendency to overdevelop one specialty in relation to others in the same medical school or hospital. For example, a university may have a very competent and aggressive professor of pediatrics whose service attracts funds from international agencies, with the understanding that the university is to provide matching funds. The result is of course that the other services suffer.

Community Health Care

Until a few years ago the activities and interests of staff and students were almost entirely limited to what went on inside the hospitals. Following a trend in many other parts of the world, considerably more emphasis is now being given to the study of community health problems in Brazil.

In order to bring students and faculty into closer contact with the community we are trying to develop demonstration areas and to link the university hospitals with regional health care centers in the rural areas. This has not been an easy task, but I think we are making considerable progress.

I was trained as a clinician and taught clinical medicine for many years. Then I looked around to see what was going on in my environment and gradually became more and more interested in community medicine. The chief problem in teaching community medicine is the lack of information about community problems in underdeveloped parts of the world.

There is a tremendous difference in what we can teach students: for teaching clinical medicine a vast amount of literature has been accumulated over the years; it has been thoroughly reviewed and valuable information is available. With community medicine, in order to teach subjects that are going to be relevant to the situation the graduate physician will work in, we need information about our own communities. But either we do not have this information or we find it so contradictory that it becomes embarrassing to try to teach it to the students.

The first step in trying to teach community medicine in underdeveloped countries is not to try to adapt information from elsewhere, as we do with clinical medicine, but to develop under medical school supervision, and in close co-operation with governmental agencies, information that will be relevant to our students.

Summary

First, because we professors of medicine in Brazil were so concerned with our own schools we failed to become involved in planning the organization and expansion of the medical school system. The new schools were established; the older schools were forced to accept more students on very short notice. If we had accepted reality perhaps we could have made better advance arrangements.

Second, because we were so involved with our medical schools, until very recently we paid little attention to developments in other units of the universities and failed to realize the advantages of association with these other components. This, of course, did not contribute toward the development of scientific research in medicine.

Finally, because we were so concerned with education we overlooked the health problems of the community at large.

In order to find more rational criteria for the preparation and utilization of health manpower, a greater appreciation of our country's needs and resources is essential. This requires an improvement in the methodology for studying human resources as applied to developing countries.

ROBERT J. GLASER
Dean
Stanford University
School of Medicine
Stanford, California

UNITED STATES

IT IS IMPORTANT at the outset to recognize that medical education in the United States, as we know it today, is in fact a relatively new enterprise. This is true despite the fact that our first medical school, which ultimately became the University of Pennsylvania School of Medicine, was founded over 200 years ago; the second school was established in New York and became the Columbia University College of Physicians and Surgeons.

Although the influence of educators from Edinburgh was strong during the initial period of medical school development, until the present century the relationship between the medical school and the university in the United States was basically in name only, even though our first two schools did ultimately become university medical schools.

I would like to emphasize that at one time or another in the course of the nineteenth century there were over 400 medical schools in the United States. Compared to the present 104 medical schools, including those now being developed, 400 was a huge number, all the more when considered in terms of the relatively low population of that period. The nineteenth-century schools were mostly proprietary enterprises started by physicians whose prime object by and large was to make money. There were those who were dedicated and wanted to do a good job educationally, but they were probably in the minority.

There were no licensing boards until the turn of the century, so anyone who wanted to practice medicine merely had to announce that

---

Robert J. Glaser graduated from Harvard Medical School in 1943 and trained in internal medicine at the Barnes Hospital, Washington University Medical Center in Saint Louis, and at the Peter Bent Brigham Hospital in Boston. In 1957 he was appointed professor of medicine and dean of the University of Colorado School of Medicine, serving concomitantly as vice president for medical affairs from 1959 to 1963. From 1963 to 1965 he was president of the Affiliated Hospitals Center in Boston and professor of social medicine at the Harvard Medical School. In 1965 he became vice president for medical affairs, dean of the medical school, and professor of medicine at Stanford University. He left Stanford as of September 1970 to assume the post of vice president of the Commonwealth Fund in New York.

he was a physician. In the early part of the nineteenth century 80 per cent of the so-called physicians had had no formal education of any kind, and only about 10 per cent were graduates of the existing schools, poor as they were. It is quite clear, therefore, that the situation then was a great deal different than it is today.

Interestingly enough, although many of the medical schools in the United States have had their "town-gown" problems with organized medicine over the past fifty years, the official body of organized medicine, the American Medical Association, was in fact founded by a group of doctors who wanted to raise the standards of medical care; they recognized that medical education had to be upgraded if medical care was to be improved.

The Nineteenth-Century Curriculum

The first attempt to set up a graded curriculum was made by Northwestern University in the middle part of the nineteenth century. The body of knowledge was of course very small, consisting of little more than anatomy and a few descriptive syndromes. Although biomedical science began to flourish on the continent in about 1850 it had very little influence on American medical education for a good many years.

There are two historical points that are worth emphasizing. One is that the Johns Hopkins University School of Medicine, founded in 1893, was the first medical school in the United States that was a university enterprise in the true sense of the word. It was the first school to require an A.B. degree of those who entered; it was the first school to have full-time faculty in a significant number; and it was the first school to emphasize the role of research. The second point about Hopkins, that is quite important in terms of history, is that it was the first medical school to have a hospital built in conjunction with it, specifically for the teaching of medical students. Teaching hospitals already existed in one form or another, of course, but the Johns Hopkins Hospital was the first one designed from the beginning to serve effectively as such.

These innovations reflected the influence of the German pattern that had impressed William H. Welch, the first dean at Hopkins, who had much to do with the school's development.

Impact of the Flexner Report

It was not until the publication of the Flexner Report in 1910 that American medical education really began to come into its own. As you know, Flexner was not a physician. Those of you who have not read this report, known as Bulletin No. 4 and titled "Medical Education in the United States and Canada,"* would find it interesting to peruse. Flexner did a masterful job of calling attention to the problems that existed in American medical schools. Some of the people who serve on present-day commissions and task forces would do well to study Flexner's presentation as a model; he certainly did not waste words and his work had a tremendous impact.

Thus within a few years of the publication of the Flexner Report most of the diploma mills went out of business and most of the medical schools that remained became much more intimately related to the universities whose names they bore. One can date the beginning of quality medical education on a significant scale in the United States to about 1910. From that point on there was a general upgrading, although medical schools continued for several decades to be fairly simple organizations by today's standards.

The Aftermath of World War II

World War II marked the point at which the character of medical schools in the United States changed significantly. The single most important factor that has influenced the development of American medical education in the past twenty-five years has been the growth of research, which in turn can be traced to the research and development efforts in medical science related to the war. Although keyed mostly to military needs this influenced all of medicine.

I would point to certain developments of that period with which we are all familiar. Although the sulfonamides had been introduced in the mid-thirties for use in certain bacterial infections, the introduction of penicillin as a therapeutic agent during the war had a far broader impact. Discovered by Fleming around 1930, the drug was a medical curiosity until 1939 when the British group (Florey, Abraham, and Chain) demonstrated its potential in the treatment of acute bacterial infections due to streptococci, pneumococci, staphylococci, etc. The drug was initially in short supply and the need for it was great. Several of us at this conference, who were involved with its evaluation in diseases such as bacterial endocarditis and syphilis, remember how precious penicillin was in the early days. For example, at Washington University in Saint Louis, where I was studying the use of penicillin in the treatment of bacterial endocarditis, we kept it in a locked vault. I

* Published by the Carnegie Foundation for the Advancement of Teaching and reprinted in 1960.

still remember that once when a nurse dropped a small amount of the drug on the floor we spent about two hours trying to figure out how to reclaim it.

Within a very short space of time, however, the drug companies, utilizing the skills of the distillery industry in which fermentation processes were carried out on a large scale, began to produce penicillin in adequate quantities. But widespread availability of the drug was important, above and beyond its tremendous impact on disease, because the penicillin story called to the attention of the American public in a dramatic way the potential of a massive research effort.

The same thing was true of work in the field of blood preservation and blood fractionation, stimulated by the high incidence of shock in battlefield injuries and the great need for maintaining blood volume in the wounded; these investigations attracted a great deal of attention. A third example of major research and development, the Manhattan Project, albeit outside of medicine, again demonstrated that given a massive effort a difficult objective can be reached. (Retrospectively, in this instance the world might well have been better had success not been achieved.) It was as a result of the examples cited, probably more than any other factor, that the American people, through their elected representatives, chose to support research on a large scale, especially in the biomedical field.

Federal Support for Research

A continual increase in research support in the United States thus occurred in the two decades following the war. In 1947 the total national expenditure for biomedical research was $85 million. In 1969 the National Institutes of Health alone had a budget of almost $1.5 billion.

The effect of these massive funds on medical education was enormous. The emphasis on expansion of research in our medical schools has had both advantages and disadvantages. Money became available for almost any reasonable project that had to do with clinical or basic research, research training, and the construction of research laboratories, and this was all to the good. But, alas, concomitant funds for education *per se* were not provided and what has in retrospect proved to be a serious imbalance has resulted. The balance of the classical triad of teaching, patient care, and research was distorted; the lack of funds to support teaching *per se* caused this vital activity to suffer. The rewards for faculty members, especially within the medical school, were almost entirely based on research accomplishment.

The situation was also influenced by the fact that support available from the N.I.H. was distributed on a categorical basis—for heart disease, cancer, and so forth. Those who administered the N.I.H. program tried to be as flexible as possible within the constraints of the enabling legislation, but the constraints were nonetheless substantial.

As a result, in planning programs medical deans and faculties were influenced strongly by the availability of funds, and they expanded those activities for which support was readily forthcoming. Consequently, in most medical schools some programs developed significantly more than others. I would be the last to give anything but praise to the research effort that was generated, because it has obviously been of great value to mankind, but we cannot fail to recognize the imbalance that has been created.

A second direct result of research expansion was that the body of knowledge grew almost exponentially, and a number of new fields came to the fore. For example, the first department of genetics in the United States was not established until early in the fifties. Now, of course, genetics permeates many areas in our medical schools. Similarly a number of other specialties developed *de novo* and existing ones took on new importance.

Postwar Curricular Revisions

Fairly soon after the war it became apparent that the curriculum, which was still very much the same as that outlined by Flexner in 1910, was out of date, although not all medical educators recognized this at the same time. The individual who deserves special credit for focusing on this problem is Dr. Joseph Wearn, who became dean of Western Reserve Medical School shortly after the war. He took advantage of an unusual situation brought about by the retirement within two or three years of twelve out of fifteen department heads in the medical school.

An outstanding group of new chairmen was appointed and a systematic study of the curriculum was undertaken. The curricular reorganization that developed emphasized integrated teaching and included the concept of free (unscheduled) time. The Western Reserve plan had a very profound influence on many medical schools, for it represented the first major effort to modify the medical curriculum in the United States since the Flexner Report. It took cognizance of the fact that medical knowledge has not only greatly expanded but that the boundaries between one subject and another were to a large degree artificial and unrealistic.

At about the same time other medical educators began to be concerned with the progressively longer span of years spent by young men and women in acquiring a medical education. Although the expansion of residency training was primarily responsible for extending the period between the start of medical school and the start of practice, some programs, notably those at Johns Hopkins, Northwestern, and Boston universities, were designed to shorten the total time by compressing the college-medical school years. They took into account the fact that (a) students were coming to college better prepared than in the past; (b) it was unrealistic to assume that students could learn everything about everything, no matter how long they stayed in school; and (c) a sound grounding in principles and in the scholarly approach could prepare the student for the continuing learning experience that is a *sine qua non* for the physician.

Interestingly enough, at the very time that some schools were shortening the span of medical education, Stanford lengthened its course from four to five years. It did so for a very special purpose, namely, to provide block time for students to have an experience in depth, primarily in research. The five-year program at Stanford in effect gave students a half-year free time in each of the first three years. (In passing I might add that we are now in the process of shortening the Stanford curriculum on an optional basis for those students interested in finishing medical school in less than five years.)

Expansion of Faculties

In the postwar period medical schools expanded their faculties; many schools had had rather small full-time faculty components in the clinical areas and depended in large measure on part-time men who derived their income from practice. As research support became available clinical expansion was often dramatic.

Some schools—Chicago, Western Reserve, Stanford, and Yale, for example—operated on the so-called strict full-time system, whereby faculty members received all their income in the form of a fixed salary. Full-time members of clinical departments saw "private" patients and charged for their services. They did not however retain professional fees, which were collected by the school and used to supplement salaries or to cover other school expenses.

Other schools operated under the geographic full-time system, whereby faculty members received relatively small base salaries but had the privilege of treating private patients in the teaching hospital and retaining the fees. But regardless of the system of remuneration the number of clinical faculty increased significantly in most schools.

At Stanford a major change occurred after the medical school was moved from San Francisco to the main university campus in Palo Alto in 1959. In a period of only ten years since then our full-time faculty has increased from about 140 to 290. Most of this expansion was, of course, made possible by research funds rather than by an increase in endowment income or any other kind of ongoing support. This same pattern obtained in many medical schools.

Currently in many medical schools in the United States there are often as many as six or eight individual departments that are larger than the whole school would have been twenty years earlier. It is not uncommon for major departments to have budgets measured in millions of dollars. I mention this to indicate that our medical schools have become major enterprises and have acquired certain problems that did not exist a few years ago. To cite one, the schools are now so large that it is difficult for one to get to know many of one's faculty colleagues.

Faculty-Student Relations

As research support grew, many faculty members who were supported on grants were obligated to spend most of their time in the laboratory and in many instances contact between faculty and students diminished. It is no secret that some schools set out to attract research "stars" by saying, "Don't worry about the students; someone else will do that. You just do your research." The size of a school's research effort thus became a status symbol.

I am oversimplifying the situation, but in my view some of the student unrest that plagues us today has resulted from what the students describe as impersonalization or dehumanization. As specialization grew, individuals came to know more and more about less and less. For the students, particularly the undergraduate medical students, the result was often a less than satisfying experience than some of us knew twenty-five or thirty years ago when there were fewer professors but they spent much of their time teaching. In that era professor and students frequently knew one another well.

In a sense the undergraduate medical student in most American schools has been pushed aside because of the growth of internship, residency, and postdoctoral programs. For example, at Stanford in the academic year 1960–61, in addition to 300 medical students there were

146 interns and residents and 80 postdoctoral fellows—a total of 226 trainees with a regular faculty of 123. In 1969–70, with more than twice as many faculty members, there are 299 interns and residents and 124 postdoctoral fellows—a total of 423—while there are still only about 300 students. Thus they are a relatively smaller component in the system.

Recent Developments

The curricular programs in our schools generally came under closer scrutiny at the time the changes already referred to were made at Western Reserve. But after a lull of some years there has been renewed interest in curricula. Some schools, including certain new ones, are still operating conventional programs, but many of them are moving toward a highly elective curriculum with many variations on this theme.

For example, the new curriculum adopted at Stanford a year ago is essentially elective and in essence allows each student to design his own program. He works under an advisory group that includes members from both the basic sciences and clinical departments, plus two students in their clinical years. The new program has much to recommend it, but to a considerable degree it is only as good as the advisory teams make it. If an advisory team fails to do its job well the student's education may well be inadequate.

Although the program is elective it is not likely that students will graduate without having had a medical clerkship or for that matter most of the clinical experiences that have been conventional in the past. They will, however, be able to avoid repetition of basic science courses they have already had in college. For example, in lieu of taking the standard course in biochemistry or histology that may cover old ground, they may take advanced courses in one or another basic science or in some clinical area. Many students are eager to get into clinical work much earlier than used to be the case, and they feel very unhappy about having to wait two or three years before they see patients. The new program makes it possible for them to gain such clinical exposure earlier.

In some ways we have come full circle from the Flexner Report. We are at a more sophisticated level than we were in 1910, but there is again much more interest in the "practical" and less in the "theoretical" than there was five or even ten years ago.

The kind of program we have adopted at Stanford, one that with variations is being adopted at a number of medical schools, has much to recommend it. It remains to be seen how well it will work. As I have suggested, its success will depend considerably on how much faculty time is given to it and how much counseling there is. It will demand more from the faculty than the old "lockstep" programs, all the more because we have moved away from a rigid grading system and from multiple examinations. How to evaluate what we do—always a problem when the curriculum is changed—is an even more difficult task.

One advantage of an elective curriculum is that change is essentially built into the system. In other words updating can go on regularly and periodic upheavals can be avoided. I am enthusiastic about this kind of approach but emphasize our need to evaluate what we are doing.

Fiscal Problems

Finally, most medical schools in the United States are currently in a perilous financial state primarily because of their dependence on the federal government. Some of our best-known schools, that are considered to be in a leadership position in terms of quality, may be in more trouble than others, simply because they have had much more research support in the past and the loss of these funds will have a greater impact.

Fifty-two state supported and forty-four privately supported schools are currently in full operation. A few of them are two-year schools, but most of them are four-year schools. There are in addition eight schools in the developmental stage, that is, they are either beginning to take students now or will be taking them in the next year.

When we refer to "private schools" we have to take into account that all of them have been getting federal aid and some are in fact receiving state funds. Case Western Reserve in Ohio, for example, is now getting a per capita subsidy from the state that is obviously helpful. The Pennsylvania and New York schools have had state aid for some time.

In California I see little chance of subsidy for Stanford or the other two private schools, because the state is already fully supporting five medical schools in the University of California system and trying to develop two more.

I am afraid that a number of our private schools will not be able to maintain that status in the next decade. A few may, but they will almost certainly need state subsidy or greater federal aid. I believe there is a place for the privately supported institution. Its independence has been one of its great assets, and I hope that at least some of our fine private institutions will be able to carry on in spite of the major problems I have described.

I am sorry to keep emphasizing dollars, because I don't think that most educators are primarily interested in money. But it takes fuel to keep a fire going and in this case dollars are the fuel. As I noted earlier, medical schools and universities in the United States have become big business. Many of our faculty members are unhappy when they see an additional person or two in the dean's or president's office; they fail to realize that when the enterprise becomes so large new personnel have to be hired.

One of our major problems is that even though our budgets have increased at a rapid rate the amount of fluid money—free money—with which to initiate new programs or to support new ventures has been practically nil. The percentage of Stanford's $21 million medical school budget available in the form of risk capital, to be spent on projects that may be of potentially great benefit to the school, is miniscule. This is a serious handicap.

We also have the problem of faculties that have been accustomed to rather generous support; individuals have related to the granting agencies almost more than to their own schools and have often been more interested in their own programs than in the welfare of the school as a whole. Most deans would agree that almost every school has some faculty members in this category, who often are professionally among the most able. Their work is good, but the magnitude of their programs may not be in the best interest of the institution as a whole, particularly at a time when funding is beginning to drop off.

We are in the process of expanding the size of our classes in response to the national need for more physicians. A significant portion of the expansion involves minority group students, most of whom need more financial support than their white counterparts. Unfortunately, however, the federal government is cutting back not only on support for research but also on support for students. The situation may well be extremely difficult in the foreseeable future.

Responsibility to the Community

We are facing, as are many other countries, the popular demand for increased medical service, which brings up the question of the university's proper role vis-à-vis the community. Some of our medical schools have indeed functioned as "ivory towers" and have eschewed service as much as possible; while we have an obligation to continue our scholarly functions, we have, inevitably, to respond to the pressing health care needs that confront us.

Some foundations have been very helpful in making possible small pilot projects directed toward new approaches to health care, but to do the job on the large scale that is necessary will take federal funding that does not exist at present. At a time when we are better prepared and more willing to respond than ever before, and when some of us have begun to realize that we are more than a little behind the times, we are unable to obtain the funds to implement our efforts.

There is much joking about the half-life of medical deans in the United States. There are many reasons why the turnover rate in the 1960's was about six times as great as in the 1950's, and among them is the fact that administrative duties have become so demanding that most administrators have no time to pursue scholarly activities or even teaching. The rewards have fallen behind the burden of the office.

The next years will be interesting, but difficult and challenging ones, for American medical education. All of us hope that despite the problems that plague us we can maintain quality while expanding enrollments and our community role.

GEORGE A. SMART
Dean
The University of Newcastle Upon Tyne
The Medical School
Newcastle Upon Tyne, England

GREAT BRITAIN

THERE ARE A FEW THINGS to be born in mind in order to understand the state of medical education in Great Britain. As universities in Britain have evolved they have often adapted themselves to meet changing circumstances. Consequently they are not logical in their structure and tend to be empirical.

Our universities are only theoretically autonomous. Each university has its own Act of Parliament which lays down its constitution; the government treasury supplies almost all funds, which are obtained by the University Grants Committee. While some pressure can be brought to bear on the universities, for example, by allowing extra funds for specific purposes, a university may refuse to accept money on these terms. Thus there is a great deal of autonomy in detailed university affairs, but broad general policy can be formulated and encouraged by the government.

In England the medical schools traditionally evolved in relation to the large hospitals in London and the provincial cities. Training was a matter of apprenticeship and attendance at medical school did not become compulsory until after the formation of the General Medical Council (G.M.C.) by an Act of Parliament in 1858. Degrees in medicine were, however, given by Oxford and Cambridge universities, where I think the training was largely theoretical. It has only been over the last 200 years or so that medical schools have become associated with and a part of the universities. In Scotland, by contrast, where the universities are much older than most in England, the medical schools were related to the universities from the earliest days.

George A. Smart received the B.Sc. in 1935 and the M.B., B.S. in 1937 from the University of Durham. He obtained the M.D. in 1939. In 1948–49 he spent a year at Harvard Medical School and the Massachusetts General Hospital as a Commonwealth fellow. He became professor of medicine at the University of Durham in 1956. At present he is professor of medicine and dean of the medical faculty at the University of Newcastle Upon Tyne. In 1952 he was elected a fellow of the Royal College of Physicians.

For the past century every medical school in Britain has been associated with both a teaching hospital and a university. The hospitals are operated by the National Health Service (not by the universities), and on their boards of governors are many nonprofessional people from the local community and representatives of the university and the hospital staff. The hospitals have a duty to provide teaching and research facilities in addition to giving service to the public.

It is very important for medical schools to be associated with universities and to have a close relationship with other faculties and general university facilities. At Newcastle, for example, the Department of Mechanical Engineering puts some of its students into the hospital each year to carry out projects such as the development of new patient-handling systems. We think such liaisons are important and they can be arranged easily in provincial centers where the links between the medical schools and the universities are close. In London, on the other hand, medical schools are much more closely related with their hospitals and may be geographically far removed from other faculties of London University. Today the University College Hospital Medical School is the only school that is physically close to a substantial part of London University.

General Medical Council's Role

The General Medical Council is responsible not only for the maintenance of professional training standards but for ethical standards also. To be legally qualified to practice medicine in Britain it is necessary to be "registered" with the G.M.C. Before it will place a physician's name on the register the G.M.C. insists on his having attained certain standards of training and on having passed certain approved examinations. It is empowered to remove from the register or to suspend for a specified length of time any doctor convicted of a felony, misdemeanor, crime or offence, or judged after due enquiry by the G.M.C.'s Disciplinary Committee to be guilty of serious professional misconduct.

When the G.M.C. was founded, medical education in Britain was in poor shape for many reasons, so it laid down very detailed specifications concerning the required courses of study and the necessary examinations to be passed. These recommendations—and "recommendations" is a polite way of putting it—had to be adhered to fairly strictly and, although they were revised every ten years, no significant changes were made until comparatively recently.

By the end of World War II people were, in fact, becoming quite dissatisfied with the rigidity that the G.M.C. imposed on the medical schools. Although theoretically they were autonomous, all medical schools had to adhere to almost identical curricula, for conforming to the recommendations allowed very little scope for innovation or experimentation.

After the war a new Act of Parliament was passed that altered the requirements for the registration of medical practitioners. It stated that after qualifying, a person had to take a one-year compulsory internship in order to obtain a degree. He was then put on a provisional register, which meant that he was legally allowed to practice under supervision in certain specified hospital posts. When he had completed that training satisfactorily the physician went on to the full register and was legally qualified to practice as a registered medical practitioner.

In 1957 the G.M.C. radically changed the form of its recommendations and laid down broad principles within which the medical schools were permitted to experiment with their curricula as much as they liked.

In 1967, when the most recent recommendations were drawn up, the G.M.C. went even further and more or less stated that medical schools were expected to experiment with their curricula. As a result the curricula in British medical schools soon may differ markedly from one school to another and are likely to become even more diverse. Currently they are still quite similar because they all derived from the recommendations imposed on them by the G.M.C. until the mid-1950's.

Admissions Procedures

In order to qualify for entrance to a university an examination called the General Certificate of Education must be taken, usually at about the age of sixteen, at the ordinary (O) level and, later, at the advanced (A) level. It is necessary to have taken a broad coverage of such subjects as mathematics, biology, physics, chemistry, English literature, history, and languages at the O level, and to have two or three subjects at the A level. Most medical faculties insist on three A-level subjects. If the student is to be exempted from the first year of medical studies and from the first professional examination, he will usually have to have had physics, chemistry, and biology.

Although these subjects were specified by the G.M.C., the universities are now freer to make changes. For example, some allow mathematics instead of physics, and a new subject called engineering science has been accepted by a number of universities.

An interesting aspect of the mathematics students—and I have learned this from interviews I have with every medical student during his first year—is that they are usually of a high intellectual caliber but more disillusioned with the basic medical science course than other students. They are discouraged by the inevitably large amount of factual material that is presented to them. They do not like to memorize data but prefer a principal or formula from which they can work things out logically. But as soon as they begin to get clinical demonstrations (and we give the students demonstrations early on), this surprisingly puts their perspective in place. Some such students cannot take it, of course, and when this becomes obvious we make arrangements to transfer them to one of the other university faculties because they are bright young people and we do not want to lose them.

In Britain at the present time there is enormous pressure to get into medical school, and all applications must now be made through the Universities' Central Council on Admissions (U.C.C.A.). The student is asked to list the six universities of his choice in his order of preference. He may vary the subject he wants to read at different universities, for example, medicine at Newcastle, and chemistry at Birmingham. The form lists the student's grades in the various O-level subjects he has taken. (He does not usually take the A-level examinations until after the application is made and the results come out about mid-August; the medical school course begins in early October.) The form also contains the school headmaster's confidential report on the student.

The U.C.C.A. sends a copy of this application to the relevant universities, and on the basis of this information each medical school makes a list of those students it thinks will be best for the school. For the 100 places at Newcastle we get over 2,000 applications, so selection is quite difficult, particularly when five other universities are listed on the form and we want the most highly qualified students for our school. If we are listed lower than third on the application we do not consider that student to begin with, because quite obviously if he is any good the schools listed ahead of us are going to want him and he will go to one of them. That of course simplifies matters for us a great deal.

Each medical school has its own method of selection and the most promising candidates are given what is known as a conditional offer. We tell them that if their A-level grades are better than average they will get a place. The grades required of females are somewhat higher than those for males because the pressure from the latter for the available places is greater. If an applicant is given more than one conditional offer he must choose which he will accept, and then both parties are bound by the agreement.

Some schools interview their most promising applicants but we seldom do so at Newcastle. Instead, during the Easter vacation we invite to the school the 120 or so students to whom we have given a conditional offer. We put them up overnight, give them a tour of the medical school and the hospital, and tell them what they may expect if they come to us. By this means we hope that we get nobody under false pretenses and that they at least have some idea of what is ahead of them.

We do still interview a few applicants; for exmaple, if there is an indication that a student has a physical disability or is unusual in some other way. We also interview all students from overseas in order to determine whether their command of the language is adequate.

Our reason for not interviewing is that under the system we had previously we analyzed and compared the grades that were given at the interview with the students' subsequent performances and found that for men there was no correlation whatever. For women there was a slight but statistically significant inverse correlation. In view of this we decided we were not spending our time very fruitfully.

The U.C.C.A. application system has reduced the costs of admissions procedures considerably. The students used to have to apply to as many as twenty-six different medical schools, whereas now they put in only one application.

Curriculum

Broadly, the medical course lasts six years. The premedical year is similar to the one in France, consisting of physics, chemistry, and biology. At the end of that time there is a professional examination, the first in the series leading to the M.B., Ch.B (Bachelor of Medicine, Bachelor of Surgery) degree.

In practice, however, with competition to get into medical school being so strong, medical schools are able to choose gifted students who have already reached the required standards in physics, chemistry, and biology before they enter. The majority of students now coming into medical school are so well qualified as to be exempt from taking the premedical year.

Nevertheless, we still want to retain that first year in order to accommodate bright students who have not taken basic science subjects in school, but who have taken the classics or history or similar subjects and have then decided to study medicine. At Newcastle, for example, we might take 100 students into the second year and 4 or 5 into the first year.

Having been exempted from the premedical year, the students begin the traditional two years of preclinical study, consisting largely of anatomy and physiology with perhaps some pharmacology and other subjects. The physiology course includes some biochemistry with reference to medicine.

At the end of two years the students take the second M.B., Ch.B.—the second professional qualifying examination. They cannot go on to the clinical part of the curriculum until they pass that examination. It is quite difficult, a sort of *pons asinorum,* and the dropout rate is higher than at any other time.

The object of having the basic sciences first is to give the students a scientific background, to enable them to think scientifically, and to apply this to the clinical work to come. But psychologically I am sure that dividing it up this way has the opposite effect, not on the best students—nobody worries about them—but on the middle-ranking and poorer students whose attitude is, "Let's get this over with. It's unpleasant but we have to get through it and then get into the hospital and do clinical work and get down to some real medicine." This is one of the points of criticism of this orthodox curriculum.

During the three years of the clinical part of the curriculum the students take courses in the paraclinical subjects—pathology, microbiology, biochemistry, and pharmacology—as well as theortical courses and lectures in medicine, surgery, psychiatry, obstetrics and gynecology, and so forth.

Elective opportunities vary considerably from one medical school to another. Under the traditional system there was no real elective time. At Newcastle in our new curriculum there is no teaching on Wednesdays throughout the first two clinical years. On that day, students may work on research projects if they wish, and there is also a three-month period when they must choose an elective course of their own. In the final year there is a period of four weeks when they may select the clinical experience they prefer from a wide range of choices.

Running parallel with these courses is the hospital experience. Before the advent of the National Health Service, the hospital experience was similar to that in France, except that all students were involved. They were given real responsibilities when they did what was called clerking on a medical ward for six months. They made notes that were part of the hospital's records and they had to present their patients to the chiefs of service when they did ward rounds. Similarly, when they spent six months as surgical dressers they had to prepare the patient for the operation and attend and assist in the operating theater.

With the coming of the National Health Service and the associated increase in the number of junior hospital staff, it was felt that students should not have responsibility for patients in quite the same way. They still attended the hospital wards but they ceased to have any effective role. Psychologically this had a poor effect on the students' morale; they felt that instead of being an asset to the clinic, it would operate better if they were not present.

When the compulsory preregistration year was introduced in 1953, the medical schools were able to become a little less insistent on producing what might be called a "safe" doctor. In other words the curriculum became less vocational and somewhat more basic. Theoretically this process will continue for some time, because very soon there is likely to be a further three years of vocational training after registration, which means that undergraduate training is undoubtedly going to be less vocational and professional and more in the way of fundamental university training.

That is a brief outline of the traditional pattern of medical education and the way it is beginning to evolve in the United Kingdom.

Curriculum Reforms at Newcastle

Major reforms in curriculum are being introduced and these can best be exemplified by outlining what we have done at Newcastle—although I would emphasize that we make some changes every year.

We first set out to define the kind of student we wished to graduate. Objectives are not usually considered very seriously, but generally speaking they can be divided into the knowledge, the skills, and the attitudes that students should have when they leave medical school. As an example of an attitude, we hope that our graduates feel that they will have to remain students all of their lives.

In 1965 the Royal (Todd) Commission on Medical Education looked into British medical education and as a result of its report it is likely that medical school curricula will crystallize into two rather separate types of patterns. One pattern suggested by the commission calls for three years of basic medical sciences and two of clinical work. The basic sciences will include a number of options, as they do in many American medical schools and in some science faculties in Britain. Each option will carry a certain number of points toward a given total the students have to reach. This will allow greater freedom of choice. Students will get a degree in human biology or medical science, or something similar, and then go on for two more years to earn the M.B. degree. In Britain the doctorate is a postgraduate degree requiring a thesis, and it may be obtained a few years after graduation.

The other type of curriculum, which we are developing at Newcastle, is a five-year course at the beginning of which strong emphasis is placed on the basic sciences, including physiology, anatomy, etc. The course tends to be integrated and profusely illustrated with clinical material at every point—students have clinical demonstrations within six weeks of entering medical school. Gradually they will get more and more clinical experience and at the same time continue to get basic science training. In other words, we would like to blur the division between "basic" sciences and clinical studies.

At Newcastle we do not believe that a degree obtained in medical science is really of much value if everyone gets it merely as a decoration for part of his normal medical course. This is particularly true if it is a sort of compensation prize for those who are not good enough to complete the entire medical course. That is hardly what the Todd Commission had in mind. An extra degree should be awarded for an extra course of study completed satisfactorily; in many medical schools, including Newcastle, students may take an extra year and earn a science degree in whatever subject they take. Traditionally, it is in either anatomy or physiology.

In addition, starting in July 1970 we will introduce a course in which students may take an extra year at various points in the curriculum and obtain a degree in medical sciences. It will be a difficult program and a core of knowledge will be required consisting largely of advanced studies in experimental design, the principles of measurement and instrumentation, the use of isotopes and computers in medicine, and so on. This will take up about one-third of the year. The other two-thirds will be devoted to an option of the student's own choice. He will be required to work on a research project and at the same time study in depth those subjects relevant to the project. In other words it will be a project-oriented rather than a formal course.

We will probably have to have another course for students who are not quite good enough to complete the whole medical course. At present we do not have many such students in our medical schools, but as enrollment increases so will the number of less-qualified students. Those that drop out of the medical course at the end of two years will take one more year in a number of subjects, including the behavioral sciences, and get a pass degree that will qualify them to go into industry, to teach, or to enter one of the professions ancillary to medicine.

Integrated Teaching at Newcastle

We have tried to integrate the teaching as much as possible; in the clinical field we have integrated theoretical teaching completely. There are no lectures in medicine, surgery, pediatrics, or any other subject, but there is a course in, for example, the cardiovascular system, in which people of all disciplines participate.

The effect of this on the curriculum and on the staff has been quite marked. First, it has removed the power of department heads to determine what is taught to the students. It is of fundamental importance to protect the student in this way at a time when all subjects are getting to be more complicated and expansive and when every specialist considers that his own subject is the single most important area of medicine.

If, for example, a pediatrician thinks the students should know about some particular aspect of cardiovascular disease in childhood, he has to make his case before physicians, surgeons, physiologists, anatomists, pathologists, and others who are fellow members of the cardiovascular system teaching committee, because they have a circumscribed amount of time, say, sixty hours, in which to decide between themselves what they should teach the students.

Furthermore, this makes the staff respect each other's disciplines a great deal more than they did in the past. The basic scientists are beginning to realize that some of the clinicians do really know something about the basic sciences, and the latter are beginning to realize that the basic sciences can help them. This is very valuable.

In the last year at Newcastle there is no formal teaching, and during this time we try to compensate for the previous disadvantage of the students having had too little clinical responsibility. Up to the final year we do not attempt to give them any responsibility; we concentrate on teaching them clinical skills. In the final year they do rotating residencies in medicine, surgery, psychiatry, pediatrics, and so forth; they are actually in residence at a hospital as part of the medical team. We allow no more than two students on a whole unit at any one time, and they look after a limited number of patients, perhaps four; this is extremely popular. Instead of being a student one day and then, after qualifying as an intern, abruptly being given the responsibility of the entire ward, he has this intermediate year when he works in many disciplines and is given duties that he feels are meaningful. It is popular subjectively—we have not yet tested its effect objectively.

The criticism of integrated teaching is that it prevents a student studying any one subject in depth and that it is far better to do a subject such as pathology in a block. It is alleged that this enables the students to study a subject in depth and be examined at the end of the course, as they are in Sweden. But this year we have some figures that enable us to compare the knowledge of students in an integrated course with those taking an orthodox nonintegrated curriculum. One part of the final examination our students take at the end of their fifth year (the next to final year) is an objective-type, multiple-choice test on the principles of medicine.

It so happened that two other universities in Britain asked us to set them an objective examination in internal medicine to be taken by students in their final year. Twenty-five questions in our test were the same as those in the examination we sent to the other universities. Our students had sat for the examination a year ahead of time, insofar as their careers were concerned, and yet the mean marks were almost identical. So far as we can tell, the factual, cognitive domain in our school is as good at the end of five years as it is at the other two schools at the end of six. I do not know whether our students will continue to improve in this respect in the final year; we have yet to test that.

Assessment of Student Performance

Continuous assessment to evaluate students is being used to a greater extent in many schools, including Newcastle. But if this is the only method of evaluation it may handicap the brilliant student who spends little time on the formal parts of the curriculum and yet performs very well in the examination. I think one has to have a combination of both systems. At the University of Birmingham, during the clinical years they have a system of continuous assessment, whereby the students are graded by each of their teachers. Only those who have not done sufficiently well in this assessment are required to sit for an examination—the top students sit for a special examination for an honors degree.

Examinations have a number of different functions, quite apart from grading a person to ascertain whether or not he is capable of going on to the next stage. A properly constructed examination will give feedback to the student, showing him where his deficiencies in knowledge lie; and it will give feedback to the faculty by showing where their deficiencies in teaching lie. Moreover, it is a very good educational "stick" to make lazy students work.

In major professional examinations in Britain we have a system of external examiners who are appointed from other universities and who, working with the internal examiners, examine the scripts of essay questions, take part in oral examinations, and in giving bedside clinical examinations. This system is supposed to keep the standards in the medical schools reasonably consistent, because an external examiner may make observations such as, for example, that the students are very weak in cardiology, and the medical school will then take steps to improve instruction in that subject. If the external examiners seem pleased with the results of the tests, it gives the faculty a subjective sense of confidence.

Looking at the system objectively, I am not sure how accurately it ensures a similarity of standards. To start with, many of the examining techniques used do not seem capable of giving reproducible results. Marking essay questions is probably the least accurate method of assessment, and in oral examinations the reproducibility seems to be appallingly low. Bedside clinical examinations are somewhat better. In the cognitive field, objective-type papers seem to be much more satisfactory. Psychometricians may be able to develop better methods to test attitudes and skills than those we use at present.

On the whole, I think that in the way we muddle through at the moment, the external examiners give us a feeling of confidence, although I do not know whether they are worth the expense involved. I think a much better method might be developed in the future.

General Practice

Roughly 30 per cent of all medical graduates go into general practice, and there is a great deal of pressure from general practitioners to train students specifically for this branch of medicine. We resist this pressure and point out that all students should take vocational postgraduate training even if they do plan to go into general practice. We also point out that we are not training a student for any particular professional role; we are training a multipotential embryo who can decide what he will do at a later date. We give him a basis and an insight into as many different branches of medicine as we can, so that he will be in a position to choose rationally.

In fact, as part of the clinical course at Newcastle the students work with general practitioners. For this purpose we selected very carefully sixteen general group practices in and around the city and gave the practitioners a university appointment carrying a small honorarium.

During a five-week attachment the students and some of the teaching staff go to the surgeries during office hours; they also go with the physicians on their rounds of the patients' homes. No more than two students are assigned to a general practitioner at any one time. The physician does not try to teach the students medicine, but he does try to show them how difficult it is to know when a person is really sick, when so many patients are coming in with trivial ailments; he also tries to give them an insight into the fundamentals of domiciliary practice.

Each student is assigned to a family so that he may observe what goes on in the home. For example, he may be assigned to a household where a mother, aged thirty, has severe rheumatoid arthritis and yet has to cope with young children, or to a home where a senile grandfather has bronchitis and there are several young children around. The student learns how to deal with such situations in the home, working with members of the social services whom he meets at the same time—social workers, health visitors, and child welfare officers. At the end of each week the group has a conference at which the student talks about his experience, the social worker describes what has been done and what remains to be done, the physician and hospital consultants give their views, and so on. While we do not propose that at the end of this period the students are qualified to go into general practice, they do understand more about what general practice means.

We have one indication that students' attitudes are changing as a result of this experience. We have now started a three-year postgraduate training course for would-be general practitioners who have finished their internships. At that time they may, of course, go into practice, but if they take the training course they are paid the same salary they would receive in a junior hospital post. Over the three-year period of the course, however, their earnings will be about £4,000 less than if they had gone directly into general practice. We had twelve applicants for the course from whom we selected seven. They have the attitude that if they are to do a proper professional job they need the appropriate training.

Two years of the course are spent on special hospital subjects that are likely to be particularly needed in general practice, such as psychiatry and dermatology. They are also taught administration and record-keeping. The course is quite comprehensive.

Statistics

The output of doctors is rising in Britain; it has increased from 3.1:10,000 population to 3.7.

At the time the Todd Report was released, medical students represented about 13½ per cent of all university students in Britain (in 1967–68 the intake was 2,544 over-all). The over-all dropout rate was between 20 and 25 per cent of the intake. I think it is a good deal less now—at Newcastle it is about 10 per cent. We try to detect those unlikely to finish the course as early as possible; in fact we believe that if a student fails in the final examination it is our fault rather than his. If we are doing our job at medical school we should have identified him earlier.

There is a higher than average dropout rate among children of physicians. In Britain, for statistical purposes, we divide social classes into five groups: Group 1 is the upper professional classes and landowners; Group 2 consists of business executives and others; Group 3 the skilled workers, clerks, etc.; Group 4 the semi-skilled; and Group 5 the unskilled workers. The highest proportion of dropouts is from Groups 1 and 2, from which most medical students are drawn. Anyone who is accepted for a university place may obtain a grant, so it is not a question of the wealthy buying their way into medical school; probably the reason for the failure to continue is that parents in the higher social classes pressure their children into higher education to a greater extent and hence more mistakes are made.

The proportion of female medical students is between 20 and 30 per cent; it differs from one school to another. Some schools in London take very few women; on the other hand the Royal Free Hospital has a high proportion of female students. We have about 30 per cent at Newcastle.

In London the ratio of full-time clinical teachers to students is 1:24; in the provinces and in Scotland it is 1:13. Part-time clinical teachers are used very extensively and most teaching hospitals have both part-time and full-time staff engaged in undergraduate clinical teaching. Some staff members may have duties in several different hospitals, however, which probably interferes with their teaching. In London 19 per cent are connected with three or more hospitals, whereas in the provinces only 2 per cent work in three or more hospitals. The pattern is completely different and arises partly from the closer proximity of hospitals in London than elsewhere.

Recently a lengthy questionnaire was sent to medical students throughout the country, and we obtained quite a lot of interesting information from the replies. For example, we asked how they evaluated various teaching methods and in response they rated them in the following order:

1. Bedside teaching
2. Reading textbooks
3. Working on the wards
4. Group discussions
5. Working in outpatient clinics
6. Integrated or topic teaching (although some students did not know what they meant by that term)
7. Clinical-pathological conferences
8. Practical classes or laboratory classes
9. Lectures
10. Research work done by students
11. Medical films
12. Writing essays for their tutors

This gives some idea of the range of popularity of various teaching methods among the students.

A. QUERIDO
Dean
University of Rotterdam
Faculty of Medicine
Rotterdam, The Netherlands

THE NETHERLANDS

THE NETHERLANDS HAS a population of 12.7 million and occupies an area of 15,800 square miles. There are no extremes of poverty or wealth, although of course there are a few wealthy individuals.

We have about 14,500 physicians—4,500 general practitioners, 6,000 specialists, and about 4,000 in other branches of medicine, such as pathology, social medicine, and insurance medicine. The physician-population ratio is about 1:870.

Infant mortality is extremely low and people live to a relatively old age. The Dutch still think it is important to have their babies at home and almost 40 per cent are delivered by midwives (which demonstrates how difficult it is to compare different systems of health care). Of the babies delivered by physicians, approximately 62 per cent are delivered in the home.

Because of the size of the country, when an emergency occurs a person is within five or less miles of a hospital. The long-standing absence of poverty and the easy access to medical care places Holland high on the list in terms of delivery of health care.

This situation makes it difficult for us to discuss improvements in medical education with the government, because they will ask to see figures that indicate poor medical care, which is not the same thing.

Andries Querido received his M.D. degree in 1935 from the University of Amsterdam Faculty of Medicine. Initially he worked in the field of experimental nutrition in Amsterdam and as a research fellow in biochemistry with Professor E. V. McCollum at the Johns Hopkins University. Later he became interested in pharmacology and experimental endocrinology. In 1949–50, as a Rockefeller fellow and honorary visiting physician he was attached to the department of medicine, section on metabolic diseases, at the Massachusetts General Hospital. While a Rockefeller visiting professor at the All India Institute of Medical Sciences in 1964 his interest was aroused in the organization of medical care. From 1965 to 1969 he was dean of the new Faculty of Medicine at the University of Rotterdam which began operations in 1966. In the fall of 1970 he was appointed professor of medicine at the University of Leiden. He is an honorary member of the Association of American Physicians.

Health Insurance

Health care is provided through a system of compulsory insurance for those with incomes up to Hfl. 12,400 (1967). The premium was then 6.8 per cent annually of which 50 per cent is paid by the employer and 50 per cent by the employee. This compulsory insurance covers 51 per cent of the population. Under the same system another 13.5 per cent of the population is included on a voluntary basis; 5.5 per cent are aged persons who pay reduced premiums. All but 3 per cent of the population is covered through other insurance systems.

Compulsory and voluntary insurance systems operate with the general practitioner as the central agency. Coverage includes all fees of general practitioners and specialists, including dentists, all hospitalization costs up to a period of one year, and charges for sanitoriums, medication, transportation, orthopedic equipment, audiological examinations, and physical therapy.

Higher Education

Every citizen is entitled to higher education after successfully completing secondary education; that is a right that nobody wants to change. Selection is frowned upon, for it is believed that one cannot provide a really good system of selection, and, furthermore, it is not possible to know what kind of an individual an eighteen-year-old will be at the age of twenty-five or thirty.

Tuition is virtually free. The university fee is about U.S.$100 and the government provides study grants, depending upon the income of the student's parents; the grants are scaled to the cost of living index. At least 50 per cent of the students receive such grants, which include living expenses, so they are able to live fairly comfortably.

Most of the universities were closed during World War II, and in the first two years after the war all teachers worked day and night in order to catch up with the educational gap. Eventually the situation returned to normal and, by 1952, with the available teachers, equipment, and space, the medical faculties could cope with from 100 to 150 first-year students.

From that time on, student enrollment began to increase, and by 1962 Rotterdam, for example, had a first-year enrollment approaching 200. In the meantime, however, new medical schools had been established at Amsterdam and Nijmegen.

In 1967 enrollment in some schools went up to 300 freshmen and in

1968 first-year enrollment in all the medical schools totaled 1,800. This year it has decreased to 1,500.

One factor that has contributed to the increased enrollment is that during the war there was a decline in the birth-rate; those born in 1946, however, would have reached the medical school entrance age of eighteen in 1964. Other factors include the rise in per capita income, the broader distribution of education to all classes of the population, and an increase in those completing secondary school.

Despite a 30 per cent dropout rate in the medical schools today (which we have tried to convince the government is very costly in terms of their investment in the schools), we still have to cope with classes of 300 students. From the standpoint of personnel and space we find we cannot handle the situation and so the battle has commenced with the government to try to establish a selection procedure.

Curriculum

The medical school curriculum has not changed fundamentally in thirty to forty years, and both faculty and students are convinced that changes are mandatory.

When the medical faculty was founded at Rotterdam in 1965, since we were starting from scratch we did make some innovations. Now the other faculties of medicine are trying to do the same thing, but under great strain, because making fundamental changes in a curriculum while there is too heavy a load of students is a very difficult undertaking.

There is nothing special about the present curriculum. It has the elements of human biology, clinical experience with increasing responsibility, and a balance between instruction and self-education.

Basically it consists of three years of preclinical courses, during which we try to introduce clinical demonstrations early on, so that the students will be aware that they are studying medicine. At the same time, we keep the basic science courses going on until the end of the medical school course, but with diminishing emphasis. There is a strong emphasis on the basic sciences in the beginning, ending up as a unit with clinical medicine; clinical medicine is taught to the students early on in small amounts that are increased toward the end.

About thirty hours a week are spent in the laboratories. We have tried to encourage more self-education by reducing instruction time and by introducing six months of electives in the third year.

In the second year and at the beginning of the third year there is an integrated course of lectures and practical laboratory work. More biochemistry is given as a block and covers endocrinology and the central nervous system. Integrated bedside blocks are also given, and diseases are handled in specific blocks.

The clinical period consists of formal lectures, small group teaching seminars, and laboratory experiences in the fourth year. This is followed by the junior clerkship. The senior clerkship carries with it greater responsibility for patient care. After six years comes the registration year.

General Practice

While the general practitioner is not yet considered a specialist, the purpose of the seventh or registration year is to train the student for general practice. Most of our medical faculty members have practices where the students can be trained. On the other hand, some of the most capable general practitioners have united in what they call a "General Practice Institute" that takes students for six months of practical experience. During that period they also receive special courses at the university in social psychiatry and other specialities. In addition there is an extra five-month internship in a major field such as pediatrics, surgery, or medicine. This comprises the training of the general practitioner.

Specialist Training

The minimum requirements for the specialties are drawn up by their respective councils. The length of the training is defined, as are the qualifications required by the service on which the training will take place.

For example, for the grade in internal medicine, certain departments are designated as A–2. A trainee cannot spend more than two years in such a department; additional years do not count. The A–5 departments are those in which a physician must study to fulfill the five-year requirement in order to qualify for his board in internal medicine.

Having completed the course the physician applies, with ratings, to a central committee whose membership includes representatives of the health service, the Ministry of Education, and the council for that specialty.

Teaching Hospitals

A major problem at present in medical education in the Netherlands is the relationship of the health service and the university. Historically, medical education in Holland has been very advanced. In the seventeenth century we innovated clinical training; in the eighteenth century it was Boerhaave who had beds brought into the medical faculty for teaching purposes. Thus over the years the university hospital developed.

Until 1940, when the health insurance system was introduced to cover the entire population, the function of the university hospital was to care for the poor; teaching was carried out in exchange for medical care. Then the insurance system was introduced and the companies negotiated agreements with the Ministry of Health on the cost of patient care in the university hospitals. They maintained that the patients rendered a service by being used for teaching purposes and that they should pay less than they would pay elsewhere. Thus the rates agreed upon were extremely low.

The university hospital has, therefore, become a regional institution giving the care that is not part of the usual package of the other hospitals. The Ministry of Education loses about 20 million guilders a year on each university hospital, because it maintains that the hospital is used for research and teaching.

An interesting point is that one large city hospital in Rotterdam was running a deficit of about 6 million guilders a year. When its designation was changed to a "university hospital" the ministry made the 6 million guilders available for "teaching and research," even though the hospital's primary concern was the delivery of health care.

The entire hospital is now manned by academic personnel from the university; the medical faculty supplies the physicians, who are paid university salaries. They could earn five or six times that amount if they practiced outside the hospital and yet they stay, and it is encouraging that they do.

If better communication can be established between the Ministry of Health and the Ministry of Education, we hope this year for the first time to work out some kind of agreement that will place the university hospitals into a general national hospital structure, so that they will be recognized as regional hospitals offering health services within the insurance system.

DANIEL BARGETON
Professor of Physiology and Assistant Dean
University of Paris
Faculty of Medicine
Paris, France

FRANCE

At the present time the entire French educational system is in a transitional state. (Actually, that is rather an understatement.)

Rather than describe the medical curriculum at length, which would probably not be very fruitful, I prefer to give a general description of the permanent character of French medical education and indicate the trends in its evolution. The period between the Debré Reform of 1958 and the events of May 1968 was relatively stable and can be taken as a starting point.

The General Scheme of Medical Education

The general scheme of our medical education system is that after secondary school the student spends a preparatory year in the faculty of sciences rather than in the medical school. It is called P.C.N. (physics, chemistry, and natural sciences) and it ends with an examination given by the faculty of sciences. (The medical school is not involved in this process.) The student may enter medical school only after passing this examination. About 50 per cent of the students pass it and those who fail are allowed to repeat it four times—twice a year for two years.

This year 26,000 students entered first-year medical school in France. At the end of the first year there is another dropout rate of 50 per cent and by the end of the third year about 30 per cent remain; after that there is almost no dropping out.

During the five years of medical school training a total of about 500 hours each year are equally divided between theoretical teaching (lec-

Daniel Bargeton received his M.D. degree from the University of Paris Faculty of Medicine in 1936 after four years' internship in Paris hospitals and one year in Berlin. He started his training in physiology as an assistant in the physiological laboratory of the Faculty of Medicine in Paris and spent one year as a fellow of the Rockefeller Foundation in the laboratory of Professor W. B. Cannon at Harvard University. He was appointed assistant professor of physiology in 1946 and head of the department in 1962. He served as an assistant dean of the Faculty of Medicine of the University of Paris from 1963 to 1969.

tures and so forth), laboratory work, and seminars of small groups of twenty-five under the direction of a tutor.

An important aspect of medical teaching in France is the part played by the teaching hospitals. Beginning in the fourth year, the students spend their mornings in the hospital and their afternoons in the school, and there is much repetition of material. An examination in each subject is given each year.

The first step in hospital training is the position of extern. Thirty to 40 per cent of the total student body are externs, students whose record in medical school is sufficiently good to enable them to take this appointment and earn a little money. They work in the hospital in the morning and continue theoretical studies in the medical school in the afternoon.

Each extern is in charge of ten or so patients and he has to keep records, make examinations, collect laboratory data, and present each case to the intern, the assistants, and the head of the department. He is a useful tool in the administration of the hospital.

About one in eighty students become interns and they are viewed as members of a very select club. The internship is a full-time appointment, and as a general rule interns have finished their theoretical studies and spend the full year at the hospital.

The next step is hospital assistant and then head of a department; between each step is a competitive examination. After five years of medical school come two or three years of study for specialization, after which an examination is given to qualify for the medical degree.

Characteristics of Medical Teaching

From this general scheme we may ascertain the permanent characteristics of French medical teaching, as well as the evolutionary trends. The most prominent characteristic is the fact that medical training is a state monopoly. All French universities are state-operated, except Lille and Angers. While they do have medical schools, they are not entitled to give degrees, which are given only by state universities.

The state monopoly has two important consequences:

1. Since it has control over degrees there is no need for a state examination; the conferring of the title M.D. gives a person full right to practice medicine.

2. Since tuition fees are purely symbolic, amounting to only a few francs, the medical schools have no private income and are entirely dependent on the state for financial support. Academic freedom is severely limited by this financial control by the state.

Clinical training in the hospital plays an outstandingly important role in medical education. All medical-clinical teaching is given in pubic hospitals (there are very few private hospitals in France), most of which are run by municipal administrations on which the hospitals depend for their funds, rather than on the state.

The exceptions are the psychiatric hospitals, which depend on departmental administrations. (I should point out that France is divided into ninety-five departments and they operate the psychiatric hospitals.) In Paris, for example, all public hospitals connected with the medical school are operated by the Administration du Assistance du Paris. The psychiatric hospitals, however, depend on the Department of the Seine.

No serious attempt has been made to evaluate objectively the country's needs in terms of physicians. The professional medical association in France is strongly in favor of limiting the intake of students, supposedly because it wishes to maintain a high code for physicians.

Much depends, however, on the kind of medical practice to which one is referring. In private practice or state medicine, better hospital organization and well-trained medical help would reduce the number of physicians needed, for many of them are now doing jobs that a good nurse or technician could do. It is important that physicians be freed from the need to perform such tasks by the training of more medical assistants, nurses, and other paramedical personnel.

Objectively speaking, there are fewer physicians in France than in Germany. If we use that as a basis for reasoning, then the number of physicians in France should be raised to the same level as in other countries in the Common Market area of Europe.

Selection of Students

Any attempt to limit the number of students entering medical school would be an excuse for the government not to increase funds for educational facilities. There are various opinions on this subject. Some feel that pressure on the government has resulted in an increase in the number of medical schools and in the stature of medicine. But this question is never treated objectively.

In contrast to the hospital career, which is rigidly controlled by very selective, competitive examinations, there is no quantitative criteria for medical school enrollment. The student is required to have the knowledge and intellectual ability to enter, but otherwise no limit is put on the number of students admitted. It does not matter if the number of students admitted is not in correlation with the facilities for education. That is the greatest difficulty in medical training in France—it can never be admitted that the number of students entering medical school should be correlated with the facilities for their training. Supposedly, the number of students enrolled, because they are presumed to be qualified, will exert pressure on the government to increase the size of the schools and to create new schools—but sometimes this pressure does not work.

In any event, there is a striking contrast between the very restricted medically aristocratic product of a selective system of successive steps of ferocious competition and the crowd of loosely selected students who eventually form the rank and file of the medical profession. This contrast was very much resented in May 1968 and was a reason for discontent among the ordinary students who aspired to a place in the medical aristocracy. I think these general characteristics are germane and more or less permanent.

Debré Reform

We must go back to the years before the Debré Reform of 1958 in order to isolate the evolutionary trends and to make a comparison with the present situation and the events of May 1968.

Before the reform, medical education was dominated by the clinical training given in hospitals starting in the first year of medical study. There was no real preclinical education, just one year of general scientific study in physics, chemistry, and the natural sciences. The basic medical sciences—anatomy, physiology, histology embryology, biochemistry and biophysics, and later bacteriology, pathologic anatomy, parasitology, etc.—were taught at the same time that clinical training was given—in the hospital in the morning and at the medical school in the afternoon.

At that time all clinical teaching in the hospitals was on a part-time basis. There were no full-time physicians in the hospitals; they worked there in the morning and spent their afternoon in private practice. The only faculty members with full-time status were teachers in the basic sciences.

The Debré Reform brought about important changes, including the placing of hospital practice on a full-time basis. Those who had functioned part-time at the time of the reform were given a choice between retaining that status or going over to full-time, but newly appointed physicians at each stage, whether assistant or departmental head, were placed on full-time status.

All new chiefs of service were to be appointed on a full-time basis and receive a double salary—one as a professor in the medical school and the other as a hospital physician. While they were not to be permitted to have a private practice, they could use hospital facilities for private patients and the fees they collected were to be paid to the hospital and put into a general fund for the improvement of hospital facilities. At the present time almost all the internists are full-time; the proportion of surgeons is much lower because they can earn more money in private practice.

Under the reform, the professor of medicine experienced a sharp decrease in income. A full-time professor now earns about 10,000 francs a month. Doctors who esteem the profession accept this because they have better working conditions, and once they are on a full-time basis they are entitled to ask for improvements in the hospital equipment.

Another change was to encourage a better relationship between clinicians and teachers in the basic sciences. Before the reform they lived in two separate worlds—the basic scientists in their laboratories and the physicians in the hospitals. There was little attempt to work together.

With the reform, basic science faculty members were given hospital responsibilities. For example, physiologists were put in charge of laboratories, or function tests, and physicists were required to supervise isotope tests. It was feared that these kinds of responsibilities would waste research time, but in fact it seems to have been more advantageous than otherwise, because as a general rule a basic scientist has only to give theoretical and technical advice in the hospital and does not do routine work.

It is very difficult to change the minds and habits of people who have been working for years under a certain system, and the effort to establish a closer working relationship between the clinical and basic science faculties has not worked out as well as had been hoped, although there are some positive results.

The scope of the basic sciences curriculum has not increased since the reform; in fact the tendency has been to reduce it in favor of including the behavioral sciences. There is a strong feeling among the students against increasing the emphasis on the basic sciences. They maintain they are not interested in research in biology. They feel they must be prepared to care for the patient as a whole and not simply treat his disease. Many of the students now in medical school will be in practice in the year 2000 and they are asking what kind of medicine will be practiced at that time.

It seems to be necessary to recycle the physician periodically after he graduates from medical school. The main task of medical education is much more important than teaching the students to remember facts and acquire knowledge—it is to build the mental mechanisms that give the physician the ability to go on learning all of his active professional life. If that is the aim, then emphasis has to be placed on the basic sciences because these are fields in which the use of logic is essential. The morphological sciences, in which memory plays a more important role, are less fit to prepare a man to go on increasing his knowledge. There is conflict then between the necessity to reduce the amount of basic sciences and the need to provide the means to continue to increase knowledge.

The Debré Reform not only affected the medical schools and hospitals but caused a profound change in the patterns of general medical education all over France.

It changed the curriculum, which had tended to copy those of the northern countries by having one preparatory year and two preclinical teaching years. It created what we call *Enseignement Dirige*—seminars of twenty-five students under the direction of a tutor. It also attempted to accomplish *Enseignement Integre,* or integrated teaching, but this has not been adequately realized to date. It seems to be a very difficult goal to attain.

Medical School Units

An effort has been made to improve teaching methods by trying to move away from the old system of lectures and to make instruction more informal, as well as to try to bring together the teaching of basic sciences with continuity of teaching. This has resulted in splitting up into smaller units the large medical schools, such as Strasbourg, that have huge numbers of students, and modeling them on what has been done in London, where one small medical school is connected with a group of hospitals, thus constituting a sound hospital-university relationship. The idea was to bring the clinicians into closer contact with basic scientists and to eliminate the necessity for students to spend part-time in the hospital and part-time in the medical school.

At the time of the events of May 1968 four such units had been completed and twelve more were being built. The units are constructed at the rate of about one a year—in Paris, for example, there will be twelve units, each with a reasonable number of students. This will lead to much better rapport between students and faculty and between people working in different fields. In a few years we expect that we will no longer have the huge body of students that we have at present.

There is no special rule for distributing the students into these smaller units. They apply on a ranked list and if they cannot get their first choice they are given their second or third choices depending upon the area in which they live. We attempted to do this by computer but it was too impartial. In order to meet special personal requirements the selection must be done by humans.

Student Riots

If these units had been completed more rapidly we might perhaps have avoided the crisis of May 1968, which was by no means unexpected. Many of us had foreseen that an explosion was inevitable under the teaching conditions that existed in the large medical schools in Paris, Strasbourg, and Marseille. But the outburst came earlier and was more violent than we had anticipated.

From May 1968 to January 1969 the students occupied the classrooms of the medical schools. The hospitals were unharmed and they never entered the laboratories, where research went on as usual. They had continuous, tumultuous meetings starting in the morning and running into the night. At the meetings they presented their ideas, some of which were very crude but constructive attempts to improve academic life, some purely Utopian, and some with too much frantic emotion. The groups included not only long-haired students but some of the best brains among the students and the teaching staff.

At the end of this very curious period the whole atmosphere settled down. The performance of the students since the revolution seems to be better. It is difficult to assess exactly how much better because we are still in a state of anarchy and there is great disorder. But there is no violence. The old systems have been overthrown and French universities are operating under provisional rule.

It is difficult to work diligently under the sign "Power to the Imagination" in a country that has been accustomed to a very rigid, highly centralized system. The French people are not accustomed to such freedom. It is like giving an automobile to a boy who does not know how to drive.

Aftermath of the Riots

The first result of the riots was that the French National Assembly voted unanimously for a Loi d'Orientation d'Enseignement Superieur

(Law for the Direction of Higher Education), a general framework laying down principles to be observed by the new universities.

The students were given the satisfaction of being granted 50 per cent representation in the elected bodies. This is somewhat of a formality, however, as the real work is done by such committees as the Pedagogic Committee, the Committee for Research, the Committee for Appointments, and so on. The students now are to be consulted on pedagogic and curriculum matters and on the way examinations are given; I must admit that, surprisingly enough, the examinations are now much more difficult than they were before. The students will not be consulted on the appointment and promotion of faculty nor about research programs.

It is too soon to draw any general conclusions as to the main results of the revolution because the new law merely states general rules to be observed under the autonomy of the university.

The second principle embodied in the law is the autonomy of the university as a reaction against the highly centralized medical education system run by the Ministry of Medical Education, and the fact that the universities have almost nothing to say about teaching methods; they only obey the ministry's orders. It is now admitted that the universities should be competitive as well as autonomous. There will be competition between them and they will conduct their own experiments in teaching methods. They will no longer be run in an identical fashion.

But the amount of real autonomy they will have is doubtful because, as I said earlier, their financial support comes entirely from the government, and whoever pays the bills is entitled to give, if not orders, at least direction.

General Trends

For the time being it is too soon to make predictions as to the future of French medical education, although some general trends seem to be clear:

1. More student participation in the administration of the university;

2. An attempt to decentralize the French medical educational system by creating smaller units;

3. A greater emphasis on behavioral sciences—sociology, psychiatry, psychology, etc.—in medical education;

4. An attempt to diminish the very large gap between the small

medical aristocracy—the product of the highly selective system in the hospitals—and the loosely selected students in the medical schools.

Steps have been taken in the direction of giving hospital responsibility to the students instead of only to externs, who in the past were selected because of their high grades in the medical school examinations. This poses some problems from a practical point of view, because some fear that the hospitals will be over-run with students. The main function of a hospital after all is the care of patients not the training of medical students.

A great many problems have yet to be solved, but in a country such as France, where the university has been very conservative and very solidified (I might say sclerosed), it is not a bad thing to be given a shock of this kind. Perhaps it is rough therapy but it will have beneficial results in the long run.

HANS SCHAEFER
Director
Physiological Institute
University of Heidelberg
Heidelberg, Germany

FEDERAL REPUBLIC OF GERMANY

A GROUP OF German experts in social medicine believes that the costs of medical care can only be expressed in terms of percentages of the social product, otherwise one always has to take into account the devaluation of the currency.

I shall try to do this for the Federal Republic of Germany and to give an extrapolation for the next ten years. The current cost of medical care covered by insurance companies for 90 per cent of the population is approximately 7 per cent of the gross total product.

The cost of maintaining high schools and schools of higher learning is 3.5 per cent of the gross social product, compared to 5.8 per cent in the United States and the Netherlands. A comparable percentage is spent on operating medical schools. This is a much lower percentage than in other major areas of the world. The figure for the Netherlands, for example, is 5.8 per cent, for the Soviet Union, 5.04, for Belgium, 4.4, and for Italy, 3.9. Germany stands at the bottom of this list.

The problems we face are, first, to define the over-all goals of medical education; and, second, to solve as best we can more or less unsolvable problems, such as adapting to the expanding role of science, and to the restricting trend of the students' learning capacity, training general practitioners at a time when medicine is becoming increasingly specialized, adapting the limited training capacity of the universities to the growing number of students who are applying for scholarships, and meeting the insistent demand of the population for more physicians.

Hans Schaefer received his M.D. in 1931 from the Faculty of Medicine of the Rheinische Friedrich-Wilhelms-Universitat in Bonn. He worked in the Department of Physiology at the university where he became a "Dozent" in 1933. In 1940 he was appointed head of the physiology department at the W. G. Kerckhoff-Institut in Bad Nauheim. In 1951 he was appointed professor and chairman of the Department of Physiology at the University of Heidelberg. He founded the Institute of Social Medicine at the University in 1963. He is a member of the Leopoldine German Academy of Researchers in Natural Sciences and of the Heidelberg Academy of Sciences, a fellow of the World Academy of Art and Science, an honorary life member of the New York Academy of Sciences, and president of the German Society of Social Medicine.

In all these considerations one must be fully aware of what I call the realization factor, that is, of the real status of education compared with the ideal that is outlined in the proposed programs. I cannot comment on this realization factor in other countries but I am frank to confess that in Germany many proposals exist only on paper and the prospect of their being realized is fairly poor.

The general problem in West Germany is that our universities are bound to tradition and cannot break away from it. They are all operated by local governments and fulfill prescriptions on a federal basis, mostly given by *bestallungsordnung*, or "the order of registration of a physician."

Unfortunately, we have no knowledge of how fully the demands for medical education are being met because most papers dealing with the subject give only estimates instead of exact information.

Medical Training

From personal experience, especially at Heidelberg where I have taught for twenty years, indications are that the value of the classic German lecture is diminishing from year to year in part because of the increasing amount of data that makes it more and more difficult to explain modern standards of medical science to the average student. This is compounded by a change in the mentality of the students, who no longer seem to have the capacity for learning that they had twenty, or even ten, years ago.

My first class at Heidelberg consisted of students who had been in the war and who had a great desire and capacity for learning. Their output was extremely high. Today when I give a lecture on, say, membrane physiology, and question the students on it the following day the results are shameful.

We are now trying to introduce multiple-choice tests which have greatly increased the efficiency of the teaching. But the students are completely opposed to this sort of supervision; they prefer to listen to a lecture and then forget it. The whole thing is a good example of the laziness of modern youth.

Training in small groups is definitely desirable and we hope to introduce it into our curriculum in the near future. At present we have two levels of training: first comes basic scientific training, followed by training that applies that information to clinical problems. In physiology, for example, the curriculum is organized so that we teach it first without respect to clinical problems, and then teach it as it may be applied to disease. We call it "pathological physiology," although the term is meaningless.

In practice, the first level is much more difficult for the student and any dropouts that do occur come after that level. The dropout rate is comparatively small—on the order of 10 per cent. The students who fail have to leave medical school and go on to study in another area (they are not even permitted to enroll in dental school). This means that a lot of time and work has been wasted on the part of both faculty and students.

The validity of examinations is very much under discussion at present. Our students favor their complete abolition and I am inclined to agree with them. I feel that examining a student, be it for minutes or hours, is not a fair basis on which to judge the results of a number of years of study. In the optimal curriculum, examinations should be replaced by a continual survey by the faculty of the capability and industry of the student.

Future Innovations

Considerable discussion has developed around the definition of educational goals. The *Wissenschaftrat* (Science Council) has tried to estimate the best system of training that can be done in the minimum amount of time with maximum efficiency. The unanimous opinion is that the careers should be split up much earlier than they are now; there should be one program for training physicians and another for training scientists in the field of theoretical medicine.

If this system is adopted, which is uncertain as of the moment, future medical students will have common instruction for the first two and one-half years and then take examinations first in biology, physics, and chemistry, and second in physiology, biochemistry, and anatomy. After this training in the natural and biological sciences, the course will be split into two or more sections. For example, the student who wants to go into physiology will not necessarily take the whole medical course, but receive only basic training in order to become familiar with the major problems in medicine; his training will be restricted to the essentials of medical science. I would very much like to see this program realized as soon as possible.

Another question is: Which areas of medicine are we going to find essential to meet the needs of the future? My ideas on this came from a simple calculation of the total cost of illness in our country—the cost of medical care, costs that arise from the diminution of the gross social product by the entire population, and the cost of pensions for the retired worker. The German worker retires at a median age of fifty-six—nine years earlier than the official age of sixty-five. By rough approximation we tried to calculate the reduction of the gross social product resulting from this early retirement and it came to between 25 and 30 per cent. This means that medicine is one of the largest economic problems in Germany. It can be attacked only if physicians have some knowledge of these processes and problems. That is why we are demanding with some urgency that such subjects as sociology, social medicine, and preventive medicine be introduced into the German curriculum.

The Association of Medical Faculties in Germany, an assembly that is constantly changing the composition of its personnel and that has no real ideas, has, under pressure from the students, finally realized that steps have to be taken. It has proposed drawing up a list of percentages of curriculum time to be devoted to various subjects. Among the "ecological" topics, for example, we would have 2 per cent social medicine, 2 per cent insurance medicine, and 2 per cent legal medicine. In total, the ecological topics would represent about 10 per cent of the material taught to the students. I think this is quite a good beginning.

Our universities need professors and students with a new mentality. I am deeply convinced that plans for reforming the universities and medical schools could be dispensed with if the professors changed their way of thinking—for then they would make the necessary improvements themselves.

Currently we are imposing by law those improvements in the medical curriculum and in the teaching of medicine that the professors are unwilling to change voluntarily, even though such changes are extremely important. I think this situation is more or less the same all over the world.

Physician-to-Population Ratio

One thing that has impressed me during this conference is the similarity between the percentage of medical students in the countries represented here. For example, 13 per cent of all students in Britain are in medical school; the percentage is about the same in Germany. We also have a similar number of physicians per population (1:620); only Israel with 1:450 has a lower ratio.

One never really knows, however, what such figures mean. In Germany, for example, we have no information on how many licensed physicians are actually in practice; not even the German Medical Association has an accurate breakdown of the composition of physicians by category. We do know that we have 43,800 practicing physicians, 25,900 of whom are doctors of first contact.

We believe that students who go into general practice should have a specific training program. An institute recently founded at Frankfurt has been charged with the responsibility of investigating the elements that should go into the training of the general practitioner.

The German Association of Medical Practitioners proposed a solution—prematurely, I believe. Under pressure from the general practitioners, it suggested raising their social standard by giving them the title of "specialist in general practice." That would be meaningless unless one has had the appropriate training, and German practitioners complain that the universities do not train them for their special needs.

We should carefully consider the needs of the general practitioner and omit all subjects that do not contribute to his useful general training. We should recognize that as a specialist he should receive postgraduate training.

Increased Applications

Only about one-third of the students who apply to the universities can be accepted. The question is whether we should expand our present universities and establish new ones or restrict the admissions. The students are very much in favor of expansion and oppose any restriction on admissions.

More and more young people are trying to improve their position in life by going into the professions. The *"sensus ministerii"* (willingness to serve) is vanishing rapidly and this is creating a complete change in social behavior as well as in the type of students going into the high schools.

Changing University Structure

I should like to comment on the changes in the official structure of our medical faculties. Unlike medical schools in the United States, our medical faculties are almost always attached to universities. Some of my colleagues have tried to change this recently because they are afraid that the other faculties of the university could enforce a change in the financial situation, particularly as it concerns the payment of fees to those doctors in private practice.

It is obviously necessary that the medical faculties should not be separated from the universities. The universities are changing greatly and some of the measures in the new constitution of the University of Heidelberg are astonishing. All decision-making bodies now have 25 per cent representation from among students, assistants, part-time professors and full-time professors. Although I am one of the founding fathers of the constitution I am not entirely happy with it. It was the result of seemingly endless discussions that went on for six months. We do not know how it will work.

The general structure of the universities is changing into the departmental system; former "institutes" in the German sense will become "departments." For example, the two institutes of physiology at Heidelberg will be unified into one department. The university now consists of a series of large departments that constitute a faculty.

The old medical faculty will be divided into four new faculties. Physiology, biochemistry, anatomy, and the history of medicine come under the Faculty of Basic Sciences; pathology, hygiene, etc. are in the Faculty of the Theoretical Topics of Medicine; then there are the Faculty of Big Clinics and the Faculty of Small Clinics. These four faculties will form a superfaculty in the future; it has no definite form at present but it is expected to develop in the next few months.

Research

One thing we are very much concerned about is freedom to carry out research. We are all demanding complete freedom in this area, although in many respects the students are against it. They say—and there is something to be said for their position—that freedom of research is inherently dangerous insofar as scientific research will get more and more expensive. A professor who decides to spend large amounts of money on a project that has no value should be prevented from doing so.

I think some ecological aspects will enter the picture, however, and they are already beginning to do so because if one needs, say, $50,000 for a project and the university is unable to supply the funds, one may apply to the *Deutsche Forschungsgemeinschaft*, the German Research Society, which will give the funds after carefully checking out the project. The people who judge such projects are well aware of the economic aspects involved. In reality, then, we do have an institution that controls research expenses and it will be strengthened in the future and enforced by the students.

A very critical point is the ethical aspect of science. Certain types of experiments are carried out all over the world that should not in fact be done because of the ethical questions involved. In Germany this ethical aspect of research will be actively supported by the students.

K. BRØCHNER-MORTENSEN
Professor of Internal Medicine
University of Copenhagen
Faculty of Medicine
Copenhagen, Denmark

DENMARK

DENMARK IS A small country with a population of slightly less than 5 million. Its three universities, founded in 1479, 1928, and 1966, respectively, have medical schools whose curriculum is fairly uniform except for minor details.

The general principles of the curriculum were laid down in 1967 by a committee consisting of full-time faculty members, other teachers, students, representatives of the Danish Medical Association, the Danish Scientific Medical Society, and the Director of the National Health Service.

The aim of Danish medical education is to ensure that students obtain a common foundation to prepare them for the subsequent specialized postgraduate training. This is considered necessary for all students, regardless of the career they decide to engage in.

Postgraduate teaching has been established to some extent and is developing rapidly, with the aim of gradually transferring the more specialized parts of the curriculum from the undergraduate to the postgraduate years.

The education committees of the medical faculties, consisting of full professors, other teachers, and students, have the responsibility of continually reviewing the curriculum, the teaching, and the examination system.

PRE-UNIVERSITY EDUCATION

In order to evaluate teaching in the medical schools it is important to have some knowledge of pre-university education. Students have

Knut Brøchner-Mortensen received his M.B. from Copenhagen University in 1931 and his M.D. in 1937. Since 1949 he has been professor of internal medicine and head of Medical Department A of the University Hospital in Copenhagen. He was dean of the medical faculty in 1956–57, a member of the Konsistorium (the senate) of the university since 1963, and chairman of the medical curriculum committee since 1961.

from twelve to fourteen years of school, the last three in what we call the gymnasium, a pre-university school. Courses at the gymnasium are divided along two main lines: linguistics and mathematics. These in turn are subdivided into various branches.

Most of these schools are state or municipally-controlled; only a few are private. The teachers have had five to eight years of university education.

The "Open Door" of the Danish University

According to law, anyone in Denmark who has passed the final gymnasium examination has the right to enter a university and to choose the course of study he or she prefers. This is a political "holy cow." The idea is that everyone should have an education in accordance with his wishes and his ability.

The number of students entering our medical schools has increased from fewer than 400 annually ten years ago to 1,200 in 1968. Of these, 700 were enrolled at the University of Copenhagen.

Some students dropout after the first few months, and only about 60 per cent pass the examination at the end of the first year. Those who fail may take it again at the end of the second year, but if they do not pass then they must leave medical school. After this initial dropout almost all go on to finish the medical course.

At present we graduate 350 students a year; in 1970 we expect to graduate over 500, and in 1975, 700 to 800.

As of December 1968 there were 7,050 active physicians in Denmark—a physician to population ratio of 1:690; within a few years that will increase to 1:500. Although I am worried about the large number of doctors being produced, it is not the prerogative of the university to decide how many doctors society should have. It is for the health authorities and the politicians to determine how many they want, and they have told us that the output should be doubled before 1980. We can tell the government how many teachers and what additional facilities we need to accomplish this task. My prediction is that enrollment will decrease, because the students are aware that an over-production of physicians is pending.

The state pays all the expenses of the universities, but they are given a fair amount of autonomy in deciding how the funds should be spent within the given budget, and complete autonomy in the selection of faculty. The hospitals have a separate budget. Medical school tuition is free and about half the students receive some support from public funds for living expenses.

The students are encouraged to carry out research and about 10 per cent do so. They have science clubs and participate in seminars and in a variety of research projects. Qualified medical students may obtain special student scholarships for research purposes. If a thesis is accepted by the faculty, a student may receive a gold medal from the university.

The Preclinical Period

In the past, the preclinical part of the medical course was followed by an examination covering all the major disciplines. The present preclinical curriculum is divided into three one-year periods, each ending with an examination (Table 1.) We plan to reduce the preclinical period to two and one-half years and, eventually, to two years, after the formal postgraduate training has been developed to cover more of the relevant theoretical bases of the various disciplines.

Table 1. The Preclinical Curriculum at the University of Copenhagen Faculty of Medicine

Discipline	Hours of teaching
Anatomy	330
Physiology and biophysics	280
Biochemistry	228
Chemistry	200
Cell and tissue biology	100
Genetics	84
Physics	72
Medical psychology	40
Introduction	5
Total	1,339

The first period includes chemistry, physics, cellular and tissue biology, genetics, statistics, and medical psychology. The second period covers anatomy and biochemistry, and the third period, physiology and biophysics.

In our new curriculum, anatomy has been reduced from 600 to 430 teaching hours, and chemistry has been reduced somewhat. Physics, especially biophysics and genetics, has been expanded. Medical psychology has been introduced.

The number of grand lectures has been decreased and will gradually be further reduced in accordance with the development of teaching facilities. Most of the teaching is to small groups of from ten to twenty students, rarely more. In the laboratory two or four students work together in groups. Much of the study is left to the students' own initiative and endeavor through homework, which is supposed to take up at least as much of their time as attendance at formal classes, which generally do not take up more than twenty to twenty-two hours a week.

The Clinical Period

The clinical part of the curriculum is divided into three periods—two one-year, and one, one-and-one-half-year periods (Table 2). The first period covers pathology, pharmacology, microbiology, and short introductory courses in medicine and surgery.

In the second year the students have clinical clerkships consisting of

Table 2. The Clinical Curriculum at the University of Copenhagen Faculty of Medicine

Discipline	Hours of teaching	Weeks of clinical clerkship
Internal medicine	225	9
Surgery	225	8
Pathology	170	
Microbiology	110	
Psychiatry	95	4
Clinical pathological conferences, etc.	90	
Pediatrics	90	4
Obstetrics and gynecology	90	4
Pharmacology	75	
Radiology	50	
Preventive medicine	45	
Dermatology and venereology	45	2
Ophthalmology	45	
Otology	45	
Forensic medicine	45	
Neurology (including neurosurgery)	30	2
Social medicine	30	
Infectious diseases	15	
Physical medicine	15	
Clinical genetics	15	
Anesthesiology	10	2
Introduction	10	
Clinical chemistry and physiology		1
Elective service		4
Total	1,570	40

nine weeks in medicine, eight weeks in surgery, four weeks each in psychiatry, pediatrics, and obstetrics and gynecology, two weeks each in dermatology and neurology, and, finally, four elective weeks in other departments or laboratories, or as assistant to a general practitioner.

In Copenhagen, in addition to the University Hospital, several large municipal hospitals receive students for clerkships, each department taking six students. Besides clinical training, more formal teaching is given by two appointed teachers in each department.

During the last one and one-half years, all students return to the University Hospital for formal teaching in various clinical disciplines, social and forensic medicine, and the final examination. The teaching in medicine and surgery is highly integrated.

The examination in the clinical disciplines is based on examination of patients; in some disciplines this is combined with written tests. Most of the examination in the theoretical disciplines consists of written tests, often a combination of an essay and multiple-choice tests.

Having passed the final examination the students are proclaimed candidates of medicine and surgery, which is considered equivalent to the American M.D. degree.

Postgraduate Education

Until recently only a one-year internship was compulsory in order for the candidate to obtain his license to practice. But starting in 1970 all candidates will be required to take a two-year internship. For those who want to go into general practice it will consist of at least six months of medicine and three months each of surgery, psychiatry, and obstetrics and gynecology. Apart from that, the course will be elective. Before qualifying to enter general practice, candidates must also take compulsory postgraduate courses in various disciplines, especially in social and preventive medicine.

Interns' salaries start at about 5,000 kroner a month (U.S. $650) and, as they become residents and senior assistants, increase to 9,000 kroner (about U.S. $1,200). When they have very heavy night work, especially in the surgical department, they receive additional stipends. All salaries are paid by the hospitals. From the beginning the interns are able to support a family.

That is the background for the rather long postgraduate clinical training undergone by general practitioners as well as by specialists. A survey made two years ago showed that the average length of a general practitioner's postgraduate training is five and one-half years, the greater part of which is spent in hospitals and the minor part assisting a general practitioner.

Until recently more than one-third of the graduates eventually went into general practice. During the last few years there has been a decline in this number, but it is the policy of the health authorities and the Danish Medical Association to maintain the well-trained general practitioner as an important element in the system, and it is expected that their number will increase during the coming years. An increasing number of physicians are establishing group practices with better facilities, better assistance from nurses and social workers, easier access to laboratories and X-ray equipment, and opportunities for consultations with specialists. A good general practitioner may have the same or even a higher income than a university professor. Furthermore, many of our students feel that in this area of medicine they have a more personal contact with patients, which they prefer.

Specialist Training

Authorization as a specialist is issued by the Ministry of the Interior on the recommendation of the Director of the National Health Service, after evaluation by a committee of physicians, which includes representatives of the scientific society of the specialty, who play a major role. No specialist examination is as yet required.

In order to obtain authorization as a specialist in internal medicine, for example, the candidate must have had: (1) two years of postgraduate basic clinical training during which surgery, medicine, and psychiatry or pediatrics are obligatory; (2) one to one and one-half years of training in related disciplines (electives may be taken in such subjects as neurology or dermatology, but many go into research in the biological sciences for one, two, or even more years); and (3) training in a department of internal medicine for at least five years, of which at least one year is spent as a resident or senior assistant in a teaching hospital attending 140 hours of formal teaching. For specialization in cardiology, two to three of the five years must be spent in a department of cardiology. The total length of the specialist's postgraduate training, therefore, is at least eight years. In addition, a great many courses are arranged by the faculties, the scientific societies, and the Danish Medical Association.

For the candidate who wishes to go into research there is a one-year elective course in the basic sciences, for which a number of research fellowships are available.

About 15 per cent of the graduates obtain the *doctor medicinae* degree five to ten years after graduation, which requires a published thesis.

Future Changes in the Curriculum

The curriculum is re-evaluated continually by the curriculum committee and its subcommittees. We all agree that medical education should be firmly based on the natural sciences, mathematics, chemistry, and physics, but the amount of time and intellectual effort a student should spend on these disciplines is a constant topic of discussion. From the almost unlimited range of scientific knowledge available, teachers can display their judgment in their choice of appropriate factual matter, but unfortunately some of them do not accept the basic fact that most of what they know is of little or no interest to the student—or anyone else.

Teaching in the basic disciplines should cover just the minimum of data necessary for an understanding of the methods and general principles of physiology, biochemistry, pharmacology, etc. that are necessary to prepare students for the clinical years. Further expansion of the curriculum should be postponed until the postgraduate phase of the students' education.

It should be emphasized that by giving too much time in the premedical education years, or in the medical curriculum, to chemistry and physics, for example, we run the risk of selecting a special group of students and keeping out a group with other qualifications—those who are interested in medical psychology and human behavior, for example.

In Denmark, as in other countries, we intend to gradually shorten the medical school course and to expand postgraduate education with formal teaching in the basic theoretical elements of the various specialties, such as the anatomy and physiology of the ear, etc.

When we planned our present curriculum there was serious discussion as to whether we should establish one or more elective lines. In view of the rapidly increasing number of students and the facilities available at that time, it was decided to adopt only one line. Discussions on the adoption of a more flexible curriculum are still going on and I think it will be possible to implement one in the near future.

One method is to allow the students to choose between a minor and a major course in each discipline and to have the minor course cover the minimum considered necessary. Another is to give the students the opportunity to leave the usual path after the preclinical period, and even during the clinical period, in order to go deeper into a special field, such as physiology, microbiology, or some other discipline, for two years, and then obtain a medical science degree that qualifies them to teach or to go into research. But the opportunity should remain open for them to return to the usual path and complete medical school if they wish to do so. I hope this system will be put into action in the near future.

Our medical technical assistants, nurses, midwives, physical therapists, laboratory technicians, X-ray technicians, and secretaries are trained in special schools, more or less connected with the major hospitals but not with the universities. Many students who fail to finish medical school become medical technical assistants, and it has been proposed that they should receive part of their training in the university medical schools. This would increase our difficulties.

Twenty years from now I think we will have a basic common curriculum of, say, three to four years, followed by highly specialized postgraduate education in anatomy, physiology, microbiology, chemistry, genetics, statistics, and so on. I believe the medical student should be exposed to all aspects of medicine early in his career in order to make it possible for him to choose between the various disciplines.

ANTONIO GALLEGO
Professor of Physiology and Biochemistry
University of Madrid
Faculty of Medicine
Madrid, Spain

SPAIN

SPAIN HAS a population of 33 million. In 1967 there were 42,000 registered physicians representing an approximate ratio of 1:785 people.

The state of Spanish medical education is almost identical to that in Italy. As a consequence of not adapting to modern trends the structure and organization of our universities have not changed since the Napoleonic era.* After many years of absolute stagnation, medical teaching in Spain is now in a period of full evolution that has come about in several stages.

PROPOSED REFORMS

In 1964 dissatisfaction with the conditions in the medical schools led to the first assessment of medical education in Spain. The teaching of medicine was examined and measures were proposed for solving the problems.

The University of Madrid medical school put forward a proposal for the reorganization of studies that was approved in 1967, coincident with steps taken by the Department of National Education to reorganize and revitalize the universities and technical schools.

Subsequently, during the academic year 1967–68, pressure from students brought about a crisis in the universities as a result of which the government changed the administration in the Ministry of Education. The new team in the Department of National Education, appointed in

---

Antonio Gallego received his M.D. degree from the University of Madrid Faculty of Medicine in 1940 and his Ph.D. in medicine in 1944. Part of his postgraduate training was taken at the Rockefeller Institute for Medical Research in New York. In 1950 he was appointed professor of physiology of Cadiz Faculty of Medicine and in 1961 he became professor and chairman of the Department of Physiology and Biochemistry at the University of Madrid medical school, a position he currently holds.

* See: Gallego, A. 1962. Medical Studies in Spain, *J. Med. Ed.* 37:892–905. Gallego, A. 1966. Medical Education in Spain, *J. Med. Ed.* 41: 658–69.

1968, announced basic reforms in the universities and in some medical schools.

In order to understand how the medical schools function at the present time it is necessary to bear in mind that the central administration of the Ministry of Education controls their finances and administration and even the appointment of rectors and deans. Any changes in curriculum must be approved by the Department of National Education. Because of this burden of state bureaucracy any change in the structure of the universities comes about slowly.

New Medical Schools

Until 1968 there were eleven medical schools in Spain; ten were controlled by the state and one by the church. Six new medical schools were founded in 1968 and the one at Barcelona began functioning in the academic year 1968–69; those at Madrid, Bilbao, Murcia, La Laguna, and Oviedo are expected to go into operation in the academic year 1969–70.

We in the universities, however, had pointed out in 1966 that the fundamental need in Spain is for better organization and utilization of the existing schools rather than for new schools. We believe that the need to relieve congestion in the old university centers carried more weight in the decision to create the new medical schools than the desire to meet the needs of medical education.

Nonetheless, the creation of the new schools does afford an opportunity to perfect the teaching of medicine in Spain, provided the planning is good and provided also that the older medical schools are reorganized and given the funds they require.

The older schools continue under the same financial and administrative system as before. The new schools have been established within so-called autonomous universities, but their autonomy is meaningless for they are also under the supervision of the Department of National Education. They have been allowed a certain amount of independence in the drawing up of their curricula, the appointment of professors, and the selection of students, but they were not well planned and they have insufficient funds at the present time. The confusion and improvisation that prevailed before they were created was such that some of them adopted without any modification the structure and curriculum of the older schools, complete with their defects.

A major problem is the selection of professors, due to the relative lack of suitable candidates and to the vested interests of the professors in the older schools, who obstruct all innovations and discourage the appointment of new professors.

Student Admissions

There is no limit to the number of students who may be admitted to medical school in Spain. Once a student has completed his secondary education and matriculated he takes a one-year pre-university course and receives the so-called "qualification for university studies." He may then enroll in a school of medicine.

Under the system in the older schools, in order to continue his medical studies a student must pass his first-year course, including general physiology, anatomy, and histology, within a maximum of five examination periods. An average of only 44 per cent pass on to the second year; the remainder repeat the first year. The dropout rate after the second year is lower, about 30 per cent. This very high percentage of failures is due to the fact that there is no proper screening process for medical school applicants. This situation is being corrected gradually.

The number of first-year students has increased considerably over the past few years (Table 1). Beginning in the academic year 1967–68 the Madrid medical school included in its curriculum a selective year with courses in physics, chemistry, mathematics, and biology. As a result registration at the school decreased (Table 2).

The new schools in Madrid and Barcelona intend to limit their first-year enrollment to 150 and to select the students on the basis of interviews as well as qualifications. Other old and new schools are moving in this direction but not all of them have yet adopted this procedure.

Table 1. First- and Second-Year Student Enrollment in Spanish Medical Schools

Academic year	First-year enrollment	Second-year enrollment	Percentage continuing
1960–61	3,827	1,395	36
1961–62	4,078	1,863	46
1962–63	4,110	1,750	43
1963–64	6,197	2,805	45
1964–65	6,600	2,692	41
1965–66	7,335	3,642	50
1966–67	7,948	3,508	44

Note: Over these seven academic years an average of 44 per cent of the students completed their first year successfully and continued on to the second year.

TABLE 2. FIRST- AND SECOND-YEAR STUDENT ENROLLMENT AT THE UNIVERSITY OF MADRID FACULTY OF MEDICINE

Academic year	Faculty of Sciences (premedical)	Faculty of Medicine		
		First-year enrollment	Second-year enrollment	Percentage continuing
1960–61	—	1,227	703	57
1961–62	—	1,124	738	65
1962–63	—	1,282	690	54
1963–64	—	1,581	673	42
1964–65	—	1,597	532	33
1965–66	—	1,504	623	41
1966–67	—	1,749	649	37
1967–68[a]	595	304 200	—	—
1968–69[b]	830	—	—	—

[a] This year marked the introduction into the curriculum of a selective year and semesters into the medical school. Of the 595 enrolled in it, 304 were admitted to the medical school in the semester of September '68–January '69, and 200 in the semester of February '69–July '69. This means that 85 per cent of the students enrolled in the premedical course continued their studies in the Faculty of Medicine the following academic year.

[b] After passing the examinations the students who were enrolled in the premedical course this year were supposed to be distributed between the old Madrid medical school (again in two semesters) and the new medical school in Madrid which will admit students in the academic year of 1969–70.

In the old medical schools, from the second year on no rigid limitations are placed on the students. They are allowed to take courses of their own choosing and many of them study under the so-called "free" plan which exempts them from attending lectures and laboratory classes. The medical schools have repeatedly requested that "free" students not be enrolled, but, although some limitations have been placed on them, the Department of National Education has failed to respond to this request. Some schools have been able to limit their enrollment—Salamanca University has almost none, and at Madrid among those registered under the old plan, "free" students have dropped from 52 per cent in 1962–63 to 6 per cent in 1967–68.

In Madrid this situation has been improved under the new plan of studies, whereby students cannot go on to the next year until they pass in all of the subjects set for the course in which they are registered. Those who fail for four successive semesters have to leave school. The new medical schools will follow this policy, but the old policy still persists in the older schools.

The total number of medical students is increasing (Table 3).

TABLE 3. TOTAL STUDENT ENROLLMENT IN SPANISH MEDICAL SCHOOLS

1955–56	15,863
1956–57	15,621
1957–58	16,592
1958–59	16,610
1959–60	15,989
1960–61	14,470
1961–62	15,117
1962–63[a]	16,758
1963–64	20,099
1964–65	19,769
1965–66	22,851
1966–67	23,723

[a] The increase in enrollment from the academic year 1962–63 is attributable to the influx of foreign students.

There are three causes for this: since 1940 male student enrollment has doubled, female student enrollment has increased tenfold, and there has been a considerable influx of foreign students.

FOREIGN STUDENT ENROLLMENT

Before 1962 very few foreign students were enrolled in our medical schools. Then they discovered that there was no limitation to enrollment and that the cost of living in Spain for a student is cheap. For example, they could live in the "Colegios Mayores," a good residence for students in the University City, for about $60 a month including full board. Some, especially North American students, came in order to avoid being drafted. In the last two years the flow has increased, especially of Arab students. Table 4 shows the distribution of foreign students in the academic year 1966–67.

In the past there were no regulations governing the admission of a foreign student provided he had a certificate qualifying him to enter university, but we had a serious problem because many of those who enrolled in medical school neither spoke nor read Spanish. This year we introduced measures requiring all foreign students to pass an examination in Spanish.

This year fifty-four foreign students applied to Madrid medical school—twenty-nine from North America and, for the first time, twenty-five from Norway. Some Moroccan students arrived too late for our examination and were sent to another school. Of the Norwegians only three or four passed the examination; the North Americans were

TABLE 4. FOREIGN STUDENT ENROLLMENT IN SPANISH MEDICAL SCHOOLS IN THE ACADEMIC YEAR 1966–67

Origin	Males	Females	Total
Europe	**76**	**21**	**97**
America	**2,607**	**368**	**2,975**
Peru	611	49	660
Puerto Rico	421	95	516
Colombia	247	22	269
Panama	193	35	228
Venezuela	176	41	217
Cuba	177	25	202
Dominican Republic	148	21	169
United States	145	22	167
Other countries	489	58	547
Africa and Asia	**430**	**12**	**442**
Jordan	166	2	168
Syria	91	—	91
Morocco	82	3	85
Lebanon	49	1	50
Other countries	42	6	48
Total	3,113	401	3,514

mostly from the New York area and their Spanish was rather good, so about 80 per cent passed.

The other reason for the increase in student enrollment is quite curious. In the 1960–61 first-year class at Madrid there were 1,200 students. In the second year this figure dropped to 700 and in the third year to 500. But suddenly in the fourth year the class increased to 700 again. At first we thought these were students transferring from other medical schools in Spain, but in analyzing the total medical school population we found that this was not the case—there was a similar increase in all medical schools in Spain. Upon investigation these turned out to be foreign students who had come to us with some credits and who had been validated by the Central Committee for studies they had completed in their own countries. Thus they skipped the first three years and went straight into the clinical years.

RECENT CHANGES IN CURRICULUM

The most important changes that have occurred recently have been in the curricula of some medical schools, for example, the new plan of studies at the old Madrid school that was sketched out in 1966 and applied in the academic year 1967–68. Starting in October, the new medical school in Madrid plans to introduce even more radical curriculum changes. The old school has introduced a system of semesters that will reduce vacation time from three to one and one-half months in order to get the maximum benefit from the academic year.

The curriculum in both Madrid schools includes a cycle of basic sciences, a cycle of clinical instruction, and a one-year rotating internship for all students. After passing an examination the graduates are given the title of *Licenciado,* which allows them to practice as so-called general practitioners. Two or more years of hospital specialization are needed to qualify as a specialist, a title that has to be granted by a medical school.

The new curriculum at the old Madrid school includes premedical studies in such subjects as physics, chemistry, biology, and mathematics, followed by five semesters of six months each in the basic sciences. During the preclinical semesters the students study biochemistry and the morphological description of the human body, followed by the functional study of the normal human, and the general study of the organism in disease.

At this point, after passing an examination the students may proceed to clinical studies for five more semesters, followed by a one-year hospital internship, or else obtain a degree in basic sciences by studying in one of the other schools of the university; in this way we obtain our bacteriologists, biochemists, physiologists, and morphologists.

In brief, under this new plan at the old Madrid school, in order to qualify as a *Licenciado* a student must spend six years in medical school and one year in a hospital. To obtain the title of "Doctor," which is needed for an academic position, the student must pass further examinations and complete a doctoral thesis that has to be approved by the medical school. This usually takes from two to four years.

The curriculum in the new Madrid school consists of one year of premedical studies in the Faculty of Sciences which includes biology, mathematics, biostatistics, physics, and chemistry. The students also take courses in social sciences and English in the Faculty of Humanities.

In the second year they study morphology and physiology and spend eighty hours on social and preventive medicine. These subjects are also developed in seminars in the following years.

The third-year curriculum includes pathology, microbiology, pharmacology, psychopathology, symptomatology, and social and preventive medicine.

In the fourth to sixth years the students spend almost all of their time in hospitals. During the two-year cycle of clinical instruction, in the first year the curriculum includes the following blocks: twelve weeks each of medicine, surgery, and pediatrics, and sixty hours of dermatology.

In the fifth year there is co-ordinated teaching of medicine, surgery, and pediatrics, and the students are introduced to obstetrics and psychiatry. There is an intensive block of social and preventive medicine associated with pediatrics.

The students spend the sixth year as hospital interns, working for twelve weeks on medical wards, twelve weeks in surgery, ten weeks in pediatrics, and eight weeks in obstetrics.

To summarize, the situation in Spain is very fluid. Ten of the old medical schools still follow the old curriculum, but they are all eagerly studying new solutions to the situation. The old Madrid school has changed its curriculum somewhat, but it is still not as radical as that in the new school, due to the obstructive efforts of some conservative professors.

The five new schools are undecided about their curricula, but since they are due to open in a few weeks they will probably begin with the old curriculum and then try to change it in the coming year.

Medical School Faculty

Official regulations were issued recently establishing full-time positions for professors and granting them substantial salary increases. Heretofore, there were very few full-time positions in our medical schools—no more than 4 or 5 per cent—and the salaries until 1960 were quite ridiculous, on the order of U.S.$1,000 a year. The increase has been given by steps, and as of last month the salary of a full-time professor had reached $6,000 to $7,000 a year. This is still too low, however, and we have difficulty filling the professorships. A new regulation has now been issued giving a further substantial increase—it will probably double the present rate.

All new professors and those in the category of *agregado,* associate professors, must be appointed on a full-time basis. Older professors will be allowed to function as before.

In the new schools the old pattern of faculty members competing for appointments has been abolished. We may now have professors, even foreigners, under contract for periods of from one to five years. This of course means that teaching has improved.

The teacher/student ratio continues to be unsatisfactory, primarily due to the financial limitations of the Department of National Education. The present national budget allocates about 10 to 12 per cent to education in general, although this year I understand there will be a substantial increase to almost 30 per cent. In terms of gross expenditure for education Spain is low on the list in Europe.

One disappointment is that a large number of Spaniards are working in the basic sciences in foreign countries, especially in the United States. We would like them to return, but the salaries and facilities that we offer are so poor that very few scientists come back.

Facilities

The failure to provide decent salaries for faculty members is paralleled by the lack of teaching facilities. Because of this, in some schools it is often necessary to teach under very difficult conditions. Frequently one professor has to lecture to a class of more than 400 students. There is a shortage of laboratory space and teaching equipment and when equipment is available departmental funds are often insufficient to cover even minimum operating expenses.

In a recent paper, Dr. Botella Llusia, the new rector of the University of Madrid, who is also professor of obstetrics at the medical school, stated that for many years there has been no planning relative to our need for classrooms, laboratories, dissection rooms, necropsy clinics, and so forth. He described the situation quantitatively and concluded that one gains a clear impression that our country is backward in its building facilities and equipment.

A step forward was taken two years ago with the erection of the new medical schools; several innovations were made in the planning of their departments and laboratories. We are now trying to find out how we can make better and more economical use of the very expensive equipment that is scattered in different areas of the schools and is in irregular use.

Social Security Administration

The Department of Health is under the control of the Ministry of the Interior, and the Social Security Administration is under that of the Ministry of Labor. Through the so-called Institut National de Prevision, the Ministry of Labor collects social security fees from workers and employers (about 80 per cent of the population); its budget is now equal to that of the Spanish government. With the decrease of private practice the Social Security Administration is in a very strong position to demand good medical care.

One very encouraging aspect of Spanish medical education is that the medical schools have entered into an arrangement with the social security agency whereby it is now responsible for the administration of some medical school clinics and hospitals. Previously funds for this purpose were made available by the Ministry of Education, whose budget is very tight.

Under this arrangement the medical schools service those insured under social security and can use them as patients for teaching purposes. In this way the incomes of the clinical teaching staff have increased sufficiently to enable them to serve full-time.

Social security also gives grants to the medical schools for research and other purposes. For example, for the year 1969–70 the Department of Physiology will receive a grant of $34,000, 95 per cent of which will be spent to augment the salaries of assistants and auxiliary staff.

I should add in summary that many of the changes I have described have been due to the pressure exerted by the Social Security Administration. They need better and more specialized physicians and 80 per cent of all physicians are now working under the system. As a result of their pressure, also, the new medical schools are starting hospitals with social security support. I can foresee the time when all of these social security hospitals will be used for the teaching of medicine.

RODOLFO PAOLETTI
Professor of Pharmacology
University of Milan
Milan, Italy

ITALY

THERE HAVE BEEN no major changes in medical education in Italy since 1861. The medical schools are very durable and very rigid. The formation of a new university is now under discussion in our parliament; it is scheduled to open in November 1971.

STUDENT POPULATION

At the present time in Italy we have twenty-five medical schools with a total student enrollment of 50,000—75 per cent male and 25 per cent female. Under the present laws students are admitted in unlimited numbers. Small universities have classes of 50 to 120 students, but those in the large cities, such as Rome and Naples, have up to 2,000 students in a class. Anyone who has passed the state examination at the end of high school is entitled to attend the university and the medical school of his choice, usually the one in the city where he lives.

There are about 850 full professors of medicine, so the ratio of teachers to students is very low—1:60—and compares very unfavorably with the ratio of a century ago when it was about 1:3. The reason is that the number of students is growing without any control, whereas the number of professors is strictly controlled by the university administrations.

PHYSICIAN POPULATION

Membership in the Italian Medical Association totals 114,000, of which 50 per cent are believed to be general practitioners. But we have the same problem as Germany, in that it is very difficult to take a

---

Rodolfo Paoletti received his M.D. degree from the University of Milan Faculty of Medicine in 1955. He took postgraduate training at the National Institute of Medical Research in the United Kingdom and at the National Institutes of Health in the United States. He is a professor of pharmacology at the University of Milan and director of the Institute of Pharmacology of the University of Cagliari. He is vice president of the Italian Heart Foundation and president of the Italian Society for Atherosclerosis.

census of general practitioners in the sense of differentiating between those who spend part-time in hospitals and those who are specialists but do not practice their specialty.

The number of doctors graduated each year is the highest of any European country—about 20 per cent more than Germany graduates with a larger population. There is a widespread belief that more physicians are needed and that the number therefore cannot be reduced. This is probably related to the fact that the paramedical professionals are very poorly trained in Italy and as a result a great many doctors are performing tasks that could be handled by nurses or technicians. The situation is not much different from that in France.

The Medical Faculty

The university structure is highly centralized and was developed according to the French system when Italy became a unified kingdom in 1861. Medical schools are part of the universities and are under the control of the Ministry of Education.

The number of full professors on medical faculties ranges from twenty in the smaller universities to sixty in the larger ones, such as Rome or Milan. Every full professor is also a department chairman or the head of one of the 900 institutes in Italy that perform research and train students. Communication among these units is sometimes very poor at the present time.

The department chairman for the past ten years has had complete autonomy in the selection of assistants and research personnel and in the organization of the teaching and research programs in his department. The chairman's prerogative in selecting his staff is an important source of dissatisfaction for another reason—in many cases his choice is based on considerations other than scientific ability; quite frequently those selected are members of his family.

The Curriculum

The curriculum is a classic one. Of the six years of medical school, three are preclinical and three are clinical; at least twenty-eight examinations must be taken during this time. As a result, the student's entire energy is spent in preparing for examinations, and he has little time to spend on research or on other school activities.

Over 50 per cent of our students fail the examinations given in the first two years of medical school, which represents a serious waste of time and money. In 1967, for example, there were 1,700 freshmen enrolled at the University of Rome. In the second year the number was reduced to 1,100, constituting a dropout rate of almost 40 per cent. In the third year only 830 students remained, or less than 50 per cent of the original enrollment.

Students must take a number of obligatory subjects each year, but few of them, particularly in the large medical schools, attend the courses. We estimate that in Rome no more than 20 per cent of the students go to lectures and demonstrations. In small universities the figure may be as high as 80 per cent.

The general philosophy behind this unsatisfactory situation is that the university was created for a limited number of students. About 10 per cent of those enrolled are called research or resident students, and they receive great care and attention for they are considered to be the gifted ones who will carry on the tradition of Italian medicine. The other 90 per cent of the students are virtually ignored. The government has become very concerned about this situation.

Teaching varies from place to place and is usually based on the block system. Each subject is given intensive treatment over a period of four to six months, after which the student goes on to another subject. In some smaller universities there is an integrated system whereby pathology and clinical subjects are taught at the same time, but this process is in a continual state of change.

At the end of the six-year medical course the students sit for the final examination, and if they pass it successfully the medical degree is granted. About twenty years ago, however, the government introduced a compulsory state medical examination. (This was considered unusual since the government controls our universities and yet it gives a special examination to verify what the government itself is doing.) The state examination is drawn up by a committee of three professors—medicine, surgery, and obstetrics and gynecology. There is a lapse of one year between graduation and the time this examination is given, during which time the students are supposed to have qualified in the three clinics. About 10 to 15 per cent fail the examination, but they may repeat it indefinitely, twice a year. Only after passing this examination are the new physicians admitted to the Italian Medical Association. This explains why, in spite of the obvious drawbacks of the system, the level of Italian medicine is not as low as it might be.

Proposed Revisions

There is a new law pending that will embody many important curriculum changes, although we do not yet know exactly how it will function. According to the draft I have seen, in order to improve teaching and research the smaller institutes will be combined into large departments, such as departments of preclinical medicine, medicine, and surgery, that will have many branches, a rotating chairman, and several full professors. The law also provides that curriculum will in large part be determined independently by each university.

The question of whether the new departments will be units of the school of medicine or of the university has not been clarified. It is quite possible that faculties of medicine and other university faculties will be abolished and that a number of departments will be substituted in their place. Single departments may have the responsibility for the Ph.D. curriculum, while several combined departments may have the responsibility for the M.D. curriculum. The introduction of the Ph.D. curriculum is a completely new concept, incidentally.

For the first time, associate and assistant professors and students will be represented on department councils and on the university governing body. The latter will consist of 30 per cent full professors, 30 per cent associate and assistant professors, 10 per cent postgraduate students, 25 per cent undergraduate students, and 5 per cent technicians. Full professors will, therefore, become the minority group on this ruling body.

Another feature of the law is that clinicians will no longer be permitted to have a private practice outside of the hospital. The law does not state what compensation they will be paid and it is not clear whether they will be able to practice in the hospital and collect fees for their services.

Unfortunately, admission to medical school will still be unlimited. As in France, political considerations make it impossible to reduce the number of student admissions.

For the first time, full professors will be admitted as full-time faculty members provided they can teach in Italian.

The law was designed by a group of five people who were selected on a very broad basis. None were physicians; they were mostly lawyers and high school teachers who are not members of Parliament nor especially interested in higher education. The group presented the law to a special committee of Parliament consisting of thirty members, four of whom are physicians and chairmen of clinics or institutions. They are now discussing the law and their first report is due before December 1970.

SERGIJE DOGAN
Dean
University of Zagreb
Faculty of Medicine
Zagreb, Yugoslavia

YUGOSLAVIA

YUGOSLAVIA, a country with a population of 20 million, differs from region to region with respect to economic, educational, and cultural standards. The first university was founded just 300 years ago in Zagreb, which at that time was part of the Austro-Hungarian kingdom. Medical education is a much more recent development; the first school of medicine opened in 1917. Today Yugoslavia has eight schools of medicine, five of which were founded since the end of World War II. A ninth school will be opened shortly.

Before the war our system of medical education was based primarily on European traditions since most of the teachers had received their training in Austria or Czechoslovakia, although some went to Italy, France, and Germany. Since the war many of our younger physicians have obtained fellowships to study in Britain, France, the United States, and the Scandinavian countries.

In the early 1950's Andrija Stampar, a prominent specialist in preventive and social medicine, and director of the School of Public Health at Zagreb, inaugurated reforms in medical education that influenced schools throughout Yugoslavia. The changes were made with the idea that medicine is not based on the biological sciences alone, but on the social sciences also, and that clinical, preventive, and social aspects should be integrated in the teaching of medicine. The number of lectures was reduced and the hours of practical work were extended. When I studied medicine at Zagreb before the war we had only a few hours of practical work. After the reform the ratio became about one-to-one for the whole curriculum; it is now one and one-quarter hours of practical work to one hour of lectures.

STUDENT ADMISSIONS

Depending upon the size of the medical school, 100 to 400 students are admitted to each one annually. An over-all total of from 1,500 to 1,800 are graduated each year, which is a much higher number than can be employed. There are 20,000 physicians in Yugoslavia at present, a ratio of 1:1,000 population, and although this ratio is not adequate to meet our health needs we do not have the funds to support a larger number.

Each year at Zagreb we accept 350 students from an applicant pool of between 1,200 and 1,400, but we will probably reduce that number in the near future, even though at present we are reluctant to take such an unpopular step. With such a large number of applicants we use a rather simple method of selection. All candidates must have had twelve years of preliminary education; in considering admission we take into account grades received in the last two years of secondary school. In addition, students must take a multiple-choice test in biology, chemistry, and physics. Candidates may get a maximum of 80 points on their secondary school grades and another 180 points on the qualifying examination. We rank them according to total number of points, cut the list to 350, and make no exceptions. Similar selection methods are used in other schools.

The prognostic value of our selection procedure for the whole group is rather low; according to our studies the prognostic value would be greatly improved if we accepted only the first 200 students on the list instead of the first 350. (By prognostic value I mean the chances of a candidate successfully completing medical school.)

We are not very happy with this method of selecting students but with such a large number of applicants it is difficult to select reliably by any other method. Some secondary schools place more emphasis on science, while others stress the humanities. This does not really matter because we evaluate the students in terms of their marks in all subjects. We look at their general education and place more importance on the ability to study than on success in a given subject.

About 45 per cent of our students come from the city of Zagreb, whose population is about 430,000; 55 per cent come from outlying areas, usually from small towns.

Before the war female student enrollment was about 20 per cent and for a number of years after the war it was 30 per cent. But since the introduction of the qualifying examination that discriminates against no one, the female student population has risen to 50 per cent. In my view women are more reliable than men, who tend to study the subjects they prefer. Women will study on a more even standard in all subjects and they often make a better impression in examinations because they express themselves more clearly. As practicing physicians they seem to have less initiative than men, but they are good coworkers.

There is no tuition charge at Yugoslavian universities and about one-third of the students receive grants to cover their other expenses. This support is on a loan basis, but good students are not required to return the money.

Curriculum

At the present time the medical course lasts five years, but few students graduate at the end of that time; the majority study five and one-half to six years. After graduation there is a compulsory one-year internship.

The first two years are preclinical. In the third year there are still more preclinical courses, together with pathology, general epidemiology, microbiology, pharmacology, pathological physiology, and some clinical courses. The final two years consist of clinical courses, preventive and social medicine, and legal medicine. The students spend one semester in each of the two years working on the wards as clinical clerks and two or three weeks in a rural health center operated by the school. Two or three weeks are also spent practicing general medicine in the city. In addition, they have seminars, conferences, and ward rounds in the two final years.

General Practice

In the past, graduate physicians went into general practice for a few years until they found a place to take a residency and specialize in some field. This strong tendency to specialize has been curtailed somewhat by introducing the specialization in general medicine. As a result the status of general practitioners has improved and many more physicians are now staying in general practice.

The Faculty and Governance

The school of medicine receives its funds from the university; half of its support is from the state budget and half from the city budget. Faculty and other staff members are elected by the medical school with no interference from outside; professors are elected every five years and junior staff every three years.

The governing body of the school consists of twenty-three members—sixteen are elected by secret ballot in the school, and seven are external members of whom two are appointed by the local parliament, one by the city council, two by the teaching staff, and two by other institutions. We may discontinue having external members because they no longer play an important role.

The faculty council consists of faculty members only, including young staff assistants. Students may attend meetings but they have no vote; they are asking for greater participation in the council. The council decides on the laws that govern the school and these are published. It also decides on salaries and promotions and confirms the election of faculty members.

Almost all the teaching staff in the medical schools are on a full-time basis. At Zagreb we have 120 professors and 230 assistant professors all of whom are full-time. There are a number of part-time instructors in clinical subjects and a few professors in graduate teaching. There are also a number of postgraduate part-time teachers in the medical school; our policy is not to have separate postgraduate schools but to hire more teachers in the medical schools as they are needed.

At Zagreb at present there are twelve postgraduate courses, each of two or more semesters. Most of the courses are in preventive medicine and public health, microbiology, medical cytology, general medicine, and laboratory techniques. Next year, courses are planned in clinical medicine, internal medicine, neurology, and psychiatry.

For a long time medical schools have been subject to criticism, especially from the health service; the most frequently heard criticism is that the schools are too isolated from the service and that the programs of study are not adequate for the future requirements of the physician.

There definitely is a need to improve teaching methods and to make improvements in the curriculum. More radical reforms are being seriously considered as a result of the student unrest of last year. The students are demanding wider participation in all university bodies and that a student be appointed as vice rector (comparable to a vice president of a university). They will probably also ask that a student vice dean be appointed in each of the schools. They want a maximum of thirty teaching hours a week, the inclusion of elective courses in the curriculum, a tutoring system, more individual consultation with teachers, and more modern teaching methods.

These demands have more or less been accepted by the university. Other more radical proposals, such as that the school should appoint teachers but that the students should select who should teach them, have been rejected.

The university has its own proposal for reforms, the main points of which are more integration at the university level, greater stress on research and postgraduate teaching, and the establishment of university departments in scientific fields. (For example, a department of physics or chemistry that would serve the whole university.) This would reduce the power of the schools and of some present chairmen, and the proposal is strongly opposed by some schools. The students support these proposed reforms.

The government sees a crucial need to reform university education, to integrate it, and to make it interdependent. According to a section of the law governing the financing of education that is now being prepared by the government, the schools of medicine would be financed through the health service, which in this way would exert greater influence on the schools' policies. We have serious objections to this section of the law, and many of our objections have been accepted by the government. It may be that the health service will have more influence on the schools than it does now, but financing of the medical schools will go through a fund for higher education in each republic.

Another item under discussion is the length of the medical school course. We had a six-year curriculum until about ten years ago when a law was passed decreasing it to five years. Most faculty members and students feel that a six-year course is more reasonable and this idea is also supported by some people in the health service and in government.

One of the most important needs, of course, is an improvement in teaching methods. We have been studying this, and a year from now we will introduce for consideration amendments to the present curriculum that will probably include the introduction of elective courses. We are inclined to introduce the so-called block system in the final two years of study, increase psychological and social aspects in the preclinical years, concentrate clerkships primarily on four or five main subjects, and so forth.

An improvement in teaching methods will require additional efforts on the part of the teachers, and this is not always forthcoming.

WLODZIMIERZ JANUSZEWICZ
Director
The Second Department of Medicine
Academy of Medicine in Warsaw
Warsaw, Poland

POLAND

IN DISCUSSING medical education in Poland it is impossible to overlook specific factors that influence medical teaching.

Before World War II there were 13,000 physicians in Poland. At the end of the war that number had been reduced to 7,000, and there was an urgent need to increase this force. At the same time the country suffered from a severe lack of medical school teachers and, in addition, laboratory and hospital facilities had been in great part destroyed. Given this situation, medical education in Poland had to start more or less from scratch.

Another factor that has influenced medical education is the character of the Public Health Service that was created in the postwar years. Its main objectives were to promote preventive medicine and universality—easy accessibility to medical treatment at no cost. At the present time about 75 per cent of the population benefits from this system. Under these new social conditions, private practice lost its importance as the main basis of medical activity.

After the war, medical teaching took place in the faculties of medicine in the universities, which came under the authority of the Ministry of Education.

In 1950 the academies of medicine came under the supervision of the Ministry of Health and in this way medical education became associated with the Public Health Service, under the common guidance of the Ministry of Health.

ADMISSIONS PROCEDURES

There are ten academies of medicine in Poland with a total enrollment of about 13,000 students. The decisive factor in the number of

---

Wlodzimierz Januszewicz received his M.D. degree from the Faculty of Medicine of the Academy of Medicine in Warsaw in 1960. Part of his postgraduate training was taken at the Columbia University College of Physicians and Surgeons in New York. In 1965 he was appointed head of the Second Department of Medicine in Warsaw and became professor of medicine in 1968. Since 1968 he has been chief editor of *Polish Cardiology*.

students that can be admitted is the number of teachers available and the size of the laboratory and clinical training facilities. Admissions remain high, however, and in the academic year 1966–67 from 181 to 272 students were admitted to each of the 10 academies. No tuition fees are charged.

The number of candidates by far exceeds the number that can be accepted. In the academic year 1968–69, for example, of the 945 candidates who applied to the Academy of Medicine in Warsaw only 200 could be accepted.

The candidates have to pass written entrance examinations in chemistry, biology, physics, and foreign languages. Their papers are anonymous and the results are evaluated by point score. The successful candidates are given individual interviews in order to evaluate their intelligence and personality. Candidates from working or peasant class families are given additional points; other points are scored for the candidates' marks during the last two years at school. This selection system is thought to be useful, although some people think it should be replaced by more objective examinations.

The increased acceptance of candidates from working and peasant families can be noted as a positive phenomenon, as can the high percentage of women in the medical schools. In the academic year 1962–63, 47 per cent of the applicants to medical school were women; in the academic year 1967–68 this percentage increased to 63. The advantage of this phenomenon is the proper utilization of talented women. On the other hand, there is the question of whether a woman can be fully involved in professional work and still fulfill her duties as a wife and mother.

Lately there has been a tendency to maintain a balance between the number of men and women admitted to medical school. In the academic year 1968–69, 50 per cent of the places were reserved for women. This will mean a limitation on the admission of women, because whereas three men have to compete for one place, six women have to vie for each opening.

The ratio of students to qualified teaching staff is 4.5:1, which seems very good but does not precisely reflect the existing situation in the basic disciplines. For example, in the Department of Physiology in the Academy of Medicine in Warsaw the ratio is over 25:1.

Curriculum

There is a worldwide trend toward increasing the amount of teaching and this is leading to a prolongation of medical studies. This trend is being observed in Poland where we have added a sixth year to the curriculum.

The reform of the medical curriculum undertaken in the academic year 1965–66 created an intermediate model between the block system and the co-ordinated system. The need for integration was particularly stressed. In that year, also, the first-year curriculum in the medical academies was reformed.

Under the new curriculum, biology, anatomy, histology, and propaedeutics of medicine are taught in the first year, together with mathematics and statistics. Thus a concentration of morphological sciences is taught in the block system. The courses in anatomy and histology are combined for the purpose of integrating these two disciplines.

In the second year the students study physiology, chemistry, biophysics, and biochemistry, and the courses are co-ordinated in such a way as to eliminate repetition—the more elementary sections preceding the more advanced ones. In addition, integrated lectures are given by specialists in the various basic sciences.

At the end of the second year the students go through a month of laboratory training.

The students' first contact with clinical disciplines takes place in the third year, with the propaedeutics of internal medicine and pediatrics. In this year they also study pharmacology, microbiology, pathophysiology, pathologic anatomy, philosophy, sociology, and psychology.

The Academy of Medicine in Kracow was the first in Poland to introduce block teaching in clinical disciplines and I will mention some of their experiences.

Under the present system of teaching internal medicine only 20 per cent of the time is devoted to lectures; the remaining time is assigned to exercises and seminars. There is a five-week clinical exercise course of five days a week, six hours a day. It must be emphasized that the lecture, exercise, and seminar on a given day deal with the same subject.

The block system introduced at Kracow demanded a buildup of existing clinical facilities which was not feasible. According to the estimate made by the academy, six hospital beds were needed for each student. The teaching hospitals did not have sufficient beds at their disposal, so co-operation with other city and district hospitals was necessary.

There is a tendency to decrease the number of students in the exercise groups as well as in the theoretical and clinical disciplines. For example, in our Department of Medicine in Warsaw no group has more than five students. The teaching of internal medicine in the course of exercises is carried out over a three-week period twice a year, with students spending two hours a day in the department. We think this is too short a time for a student to spend with patients. We in Warsaw would like to see the academy introduce the block system of teaching in internal medicine, because the existing system is not sufficient for our needs.

Particular emphasis is placed on teaching social medicine. The primary purpose is to illustrate the social components in the case of disease and the social consequences thereof. Among other things, the students are taught in the Department of Hygiene and Social Medicine during the fourth and sixth years.

In general, the amount of time given over to lectures is being reduced, while practical exercises are being emphasized. The character of the lectures is also being changed. Clinical lectures are often integrated, with various specialists lecturing. This enables us to present some problems as a whole and thus to cope with the habit of pigeonholing. Every year in our department a few students themselves deliver lectures. In spite of some criticism it is the general belief that the lecture in its new shape is a valuable tool in teaching. To augment the lectures, audio-visual aids have been introduced on a larger scale.

Progress in the teaching of the basic sciences demands modern equipment, but despite the strong effort made in this direction by the government we still have a serious shortage of equipment; clinical training facilities are also not satisfactory at the present time.

Recently, pedagogical councils were established in each year of medical school, with the teaching staff acting as tutors. The purpose of the councils is to collaborate closely with the dean in setting up adequate teaching programs. The authorities of the academies and the teaching staff are particularly interested in these councils.

There is a widespread feeling in Poland that the medical curriculum must be changed and that new methods of teaching and of learning must be adopted.

Evaluation

There has been a great deal of discussion of how to evaluate the knowledge that students have gained during their years at medical school. In general the examination is regarded as being more objective than other methods but it has not been universally accepted in Poland as yet; at Warsaw, for example, examinations are given by eight clinics.

We think they could be a very important means for comparing the results of teaching in different medical schools in Poland.

Students' Research

Students are encouraged to carry out research early in their medical school studies. For several years they have been active in a number of scientific societies in theoretical and clinical disciplines. The individual society usually has twenty to thirty members, with a senior student acting as its secretary. The societies are sponsored by an experienced member of the teaching staff. They are all affiliated with the Association of Students' Scientific Societies which is sponsored by a professor appointed by the president of the Academy of Medicine. The association organizes an annual scientific conference at which the results of the most successful research projects are presented.

Student members of the societies carry on research and prepare lectures to be given and discussed at the regular meetings. It is generally believed that future scientific workers will evolve from these associations.

J. S. W. LUTWAMA
Dean
Makerere University College
Faculty of Medicine
Kampala, Uganda

EAST AFRICA

The importance in medical education of taking into account local health requirements cannot be overemphasized. Progressive medical schools all over the world are revising their undergraduate and postgraduate training programs and adapting them to local or regional health requirements.

In East Africa, in collaboration with the ministries of health and education in Uganda, Kenya, and Tanzania, the East African Association of Physicians and Surgeons and the East African Council for Medical Education, Makerere medical school has played a leading role in this connection.

For example, the undergraduate curriculum was revised in 1963 and again in 1966, and postgraduate training programs specifically designed to produce badly needed specialists and medical teachers were inaugurated in 1967 (see Appendices 1, 2, and 3).

Educational Objectives

Unambiguous educational objectives defined in behavioral terms are essential for the evaluation of any medical education program. At the first meeting of professors of public health in the African regions, held in Brazaville in 1968, Dr. J. J. Guilbert, Education and Training Advisor in the World Health Organization Regional Office for Africa, stated correctly and in the clearest possible language:

Joseph S. W. Lutwama obtained his L.M.S. (Licentiateship in Medicine and Surgery) in 1956 and the M.B., Ch.B. in 1964, both in East Africa. In 1965 he was elected professor of preventive medicine and dean of the Faculty of Medicine at Makerere University College, University of East Africa. He held these posts until December 1969 when he was appointed full-time dean and director of postgraduate medical studies. He served as president of the Association of Medical Schools in Africa from 1967 to 1969 and as chairman of the East African Council for Medical Education from 1965 to 1969. Dean Lutwama's other degrees include Diploma in Public Health (St. Andrew's), Diploma in Child Health (London), Diploma in Advanced Maternal and Child Health (Uppsala), and Diploma in Industrial Health (St. Andrew's). He is a M.R.C.P. (Dublin) and a F.R.S.M. (London).

The educational goals must be defined by using *behavioral terms* corresponding to the task to be accomplished. In other words, the definition must indicate *what the graduates of a given school will be able to DO at the end of their period of education or training that they were not able to do before.*

This is a very difficult task which may well have daunted the most conscientious. We consider that assistance in this field should be given to teachers in the form of written documents, seminars, etc.

The lack of any definition of educational goals makes discussions on programs, teaching methods, and evaluation methods completely vain and futile.

Evaluation methods can be selected only in terms of the objectives to be attained. Evaluation consists of being able to say to what *measurable* extent the assigned objective has been attained. If one has not taken the trouble to establish a *measurable* objective it is impossible to make any kind of evaluation.

The tasks corresponding to the educational objectives to be defined must, of course, be related to the major health problems—physical, mental, and social—of the community and to the basic health services, namely: health education; maternal and child health; communicable disease control; environmental sanitation; maintenance of records for statistical purposes; public health nursing; and medical care (including, of course, curative services).

Special attention must be paid to the system for the delivery of health care. Medical personnel who have undergone excellent training will be unable to "deliver the goods" unless there is a reasonable system for delivering health care to all segments of the community. Educational goals as suggested in the foregoing must be *feasible, observable,* and *measurable.*

Major Advances in East Africa

Undergraduate Medical Education

The new curriculum introduced at Makerere medical school in July 1963 represented a major step forward. Prior to that time medical educators in East Africa, although acutely aware of the great need for a curriculum geared to specific African health problems, were reluctant to introduce major changes in the curriculum for fear that the General Medical Council of Great Britain would withdraw recognition of the East African medical qualification. Events since 1963 have shown that such fears were unfounded. Increasingly, medical educators in the developing countries, including East Africa, have stopped regarding "international recognition" as an end in itself.

The students who were admitted under the first year of the new curriculum took the final M.B., Ch.B. degree examination in March 1968 with very gratifying results. Examiners from other universities in Africa and from Britain were very much impressed with the outcome of this experiment. Even better results are expected from yet another new curriculum that was adopted in July 1966 (see Appendix 1).

Concurrently, some exciting developments are taking place at Dar es Salaam University College Medical School, where a new curriculum has been introduced that differs significantly from the traditional curricula (see Appendix 2).

Postgraduate Medical Education (see Appendix 3)

The inauguration in 1967 of the Master of Medicine (M.Med.) postgraduate, residency-type training programs at Makerere was a most important event. It clearly demonstrated that the University of East Africa, with the full support of the three East African governments, had assumed the responsibility for the postgraduate training of badly needed specialists and medical school teachers. The degree of M.Med. in medicine, surgery, obstetrics and gynecology, pediatrics, psychiatry, public health, and pathology, respectively, is designed as a specialist professional qualification at least equivalent to the postgraduate diplomas awarded by the royal colleges in Britain (for example the M.R.C.P., M.R.C.O.G., and F.R.C.S.) or to the state specialty board certification in the United States.

The first and historic M.Med. degree examinations will be held at Makerere in March 1970. Examiners from other African medical schools, from Britain, and possibly from North America, will participate. There is little doubt that this East African program will be of great interest to other countries, particularly to the developing countries, where the faculties of medicine are the only bodies equipped to supervise postgraduate medical education.

In July 1967 the first course in Middle Africa leading to a doctorate in public health was launched successfully at Makerere, with one student from Nigeria and four from Uganda. The second course was started in July 1968, with two students from Kenya, two from Uganda, one from Zambia, and one from Britain (the English wife of an American staff member). In the third course, which began in July 1969, there were two students each from Uganda, Kenya, Tanzania, and Nigeria. Six of the students are on W.H.O. fellowships. Needless to say, this

D.P.H. course has been geared to African public health problems and will be kept under continuous review in the light of feedback from the students and advice from colleagues at other medical schools in Africa.

Before 1967, doctors requiring postgraduate training in public health were sent to Britain and North America to obtain the D.P.H. or M.P.H. degree. It is most likely that courses leading to the diploma in tropical public health that are conducted in temperate zone countries will become less and less fashionable.

Assessment of Requirements for Training and Education

By the 1980's the arbitrary aim is to provide one physician for each 10,000 population in East Africa. The crude needs are estimated in Table 1, which shows population projections for urban and rural areas in Kenya, Uganda, and Tanzania.

Medical Schools and Teaching Hospitals

In order to meet the proposed physician:population ratio by the 1980's, 3 schools would each have to produce 100 doctors each year, beginning in the early 1970's. In order to reach this figure an early expansion is necessary of the medical schools at both Nairobi and Dar es Salaam, but even then there will be a gap, for such an annual output could not be reached until the mid-1970's.

The creation of a fourth medical school in the early 1970's is highly desirable due to the public demand for better service and less dependence on auxiliaries, especially in the urban areas, and unanimous agreement that health services should become less dependent on a cosmopolitan assortment of short-term, expatriate doctors. A sufficient output of suitable medical school candidates from the secondary schools would justify this further expansion.

Medical School Staff

At present a medical school of the size of Makerere is staffed by approximately twenty preclinical teachers, fifteen paraclinical teachers and five honorary paraclinical teachers, and forty-five clinical teachers and forty-five honorary clinical teachers.

Thus within the next three to five years three medical schools would need sixty preclinical teachers (seventy, if schools of dentistry and pharmacy are established), sixty paraclinical teachers, and 280 clinical teachers. Currently only about 20 to 30 per cent of medical school teachers are East Africans.

TABLE 1. CURRENT AND PROJECTED REQUIREMENTS OF MEDICAL MANPOWER IN EAST AFRICA[a] (IN HUNDREDS OF THOUSANDS)

	Estimated 1970 population of East Africa				Projected 1980 population of East Africa			
	Kenya	Uganda	Tanzania	Total	Kenya	Uganda	Tanzania	Total
Urban	1,086	567	731	2,384	1,772	953	1,221	3,946
Rural	9,761	7,972	10,519	28,252	12,750	9,965	12,887	35,602
Total	10,847	8,539	11,250	30,636	14,522	10,918	14,108	39,548
Number of doctors needed[b]	1,084	854	1,125	3,063	1,452	1,092	1,411	3,955

[a] Based on a paper by Bennett, F. J., Hall, S. A., Lutwama, J. S. W., and Rado, E. R. 1965. Medical Manpower in East Africa, Prospects and Problems, *E.A.M.J.* 42:4.

[b] On the basis of 1:10,000 population.

Requirements for Specialists and Other Practitioners

Since it is estimated that from 85 to 95 per cent of the populations will still live in the rural areas in the 1980's, the developing pattern of medical care in these areas is to have health centers operated by medical auxiliaries. They will be connected with a network of regional or subregional (larger district) hospitals staffed by specialists—there will be one such hospital per 1 million population. By 1980 about forty of these hospitals will be needed in East Africa, each being staffed by eight clinical specialists (medicine, surgery [orthopedic, ophthalmic, ENT], obstetrics and gynecology, pediatrics, mental health, etc.)—a total requirement of about 320 clinical specialists.

The growth of towns may be accompanied by a move toward group practice with perhaps pediatric and obstetric specialists (or diplomates) being associated with such groups. Assuming the attachment of only two specialists to each of fifty urban general group practices (perhaps too conservative an estimate) this would require another 100 private specialists in East Africa.

Some industries might sponsor group occupational health services, as they are already doing in Nairobi and Dar es Salaam, and this would call for perhaps twenty practitioners with a degree in industrial health medicine by 1980.

At the present time the private-physician-to-city-dweller ratio is 1:2,000. In East Africa by 1980 there will be approximately 4 million people in the cities; assuming the ratio remains the same, 2,000 private practitioners would be required—an increase of about 1,300 over the present level of 700; (they should really be calculated separately from the demand for an over-all ratio of 1:10,000 population). It is open for consideration whether these 1,300 private practitioners will be drawn from privately financed or other graduates of East African medical schools, who will become attracted by the rewards that uncontrolled free enterprise practice will provide in a growing urban population where the fees for medical care obviously relate to the demand, or from expatriates who will be attracted by the possibilities, or from both sources.

Summary of Requirements

To meet the conservative estimate of the needs of the 1980's will require three medical schools each graduating 100 doctors a year. A first priority is to raise the output of all three schools to this level. Reasons have been advanced for the establishment of a fourth school in the 1970's.

The expansion of medical school faculties (on which East Africans are currently underrepresented) and of the network of regional hospitals with staff specialists will make it necessary by 1980 to have approximately 400 teachers in the three medical schools and a further 320 specialists in the principal clinical disciplines to man the regional hospitals. Even if only 60 per cent, or 240, of the teaching staff were East African graduates this would entail a training program for almost 550 specialists over the next twelve to thirteen years, that is, around 40 to 45 each year—perhaps 10 to 12 in each of the main clinical disciplines of medicine, surgery, pediatrics, and obstetrics and gynecology. In addition there will be the less predictable demand for specialists from the private sector.

The field of public health may be considered separately. The demand will be primarily for physicians with postgraduate qualifications to serve as district medical officers (or district consultants in preventive medicine) and other miscellaneous posts in administration, laboratories, and research facilities. This would call for eighty posts to be filled in the next twelve years and require an average output of six to seven doctors of public health a year.

The foregoing estimates are by no means extravagant and demonstrate quite clearly that the problem of satisfying East Africa's requirements for high-level medical teachers and specialists is gigantic and calls for meticulous planning and the pooling of resources on a regional basis. Expanded M.Med. and D.P.H. training programs provide the best hope of satisfying these requirements. External assistance in the development of well-equipped regional centers for postgraduate medical education would be invaluable and would produce lasting results beyond all expectations.

APPENDIX 1
Makerere University College Faculty of Medicine Undergraduate Curriculum

Introduction

During the developmental period of the medical school toward full university status, from 1950 to 1960, the curriculum was based essentially on the London M.B., B.S. pattern. This consisted of two years, each of three terms, devoted to anatomy, physiology, and biochemistry. There was a long vacation in each of these years. There followed three years of clinical work in which little preventive medicine or pediatrics was included.

In 1960 it was decided to revise the curriculum in order to make it more relevant to conditions in East Africa. At that time there was an average admission of twenty students a year into the medical school and it was predicted that there would be a gradual increase to sixty admissions in 1970.

The new curriculum was introduced in 1963. In it, anatomy, physiology, and biochemistry were compressed into one four-term year. There was a two-term introductory course in year two, followed by two terms of clerking in medicine and surgery. It was envisaged that additional anatomy and physiology would be taught during the clinical course. Years three and four consisted of only three terms of clerking followed by long vacations at the end of each. Preventive medicine and pediatrics received a larger share of the clerking period, with obstetrics, gynecology, medical and surgical "specials" forming the other four clerking periods in these two years. Year five consisted of a second clerkship in medicine and surgery followed by a revision term.

Shortly after this curriculum was introduced radical changes were made in both the rate and size of the medical school's development; an intake of ninety students was expected in 1966 and it was believed that such an increase would continue indefinitely.

At this point it became evident that our new curriculum, planned around a smaller number of students, was not going to be successful. In the first place, with a rather variable Higher School Certificate entry level it was proving very difficult to cover all the basic sciences adequately in one year, particularly with a decrease in the opportunities for contact between the staff and the students. This resulted in students arriving at their clerkship periods with insufficient knowledge of the basic sciences.

Second, the large number of students made it impossible for clerking to be done on a small-group basis, which is the keystone of clinical teaching. Furthermore, from the end of March until the beginning of July there were virtually no students in the hospital.

By 1966, therefore, it became evident to the Curriculum Committee that we would have to alter the curriculum again to meet the changed situation. Two fundamental criteria would have to be met: the first was the need to allow more time to the basic medical sciences to prepare the students for their introduction to clinical work; the second was the need to use the hospital throughout the academic year. In this way ninety students could be split into four groups instead of three and thus receive more individual attention.

In the final planning of the present curriculum we were also influenced by the age structure and disease pattern of the population and by the socioeconomic cultural patterns and organization of medical practice in East Africa. We were also determined to try to attain a more genuine integration of subject matter instead of the rather pseudointegration in the previous curriculum.

General Outline of the Present Curriculum

Although the curriculum has been designed as a unified course, for the present purposes it can be divided into two parts:

1. The first two years (each consisting of four terms of ten weeks) are spent preparing the student in the basic sciences. During this time he learns about the normal structure and function of the body from the level of the smallest cell organelle to the complex structure and control of systems such as the central nervous system. He also learns about the normal development of man in terms of his behavior and psychological interaction with other individuals. He gains practical experience in physiological, biochemical, and other techniques and a course in statistics enables him to appreciate the significance of experimental results.

In the second year the student is introduced to the causes of disease and to the abnormalities of structure and function that result therefrom. These general principles of pathology and microbiology are illustrated by a series of clinicopathological sessions. Medical genetics, medical immunology, and the history of medicine are taught as interdepartmental subjects; the general principles of epidemiology illustrate community aspects of disease. The basis of drug action and therapeutic principles are also given during this period.

2. During the next three years the student learns the practice of medicine in the widest sense. In year three he spends four terms attached in turn to the departments of medicine, surgery, obstetrics and gynecology, and pediatrics. Instruction on the wards, with patient attachment, forms the basis of these clerkships and the student is expected to become familiar with simple technical procedures in the ward and laboratory. An integrated lecture-seminar course on systemic disease is given in which all clinical and paraclinical departments take part. Conjoint seminars, grand rounds, slide seminars, and autopsy demonstrations continue throughout this period. The importance of community medicine and preventive medicine are stressed by co-operative sessions with the Department of Preventive Medicine.

At the beginning of the fourth year the students have a long vacation during which it is hoped that many of them will carry on an elective study or a research project. In the fourth year practical instruction is given and clinical experience is obtained in a five-week clerkship in psychiatry. A further five-week attachment to the Department of Preventive Medicine with work at Kasangati Rural Health Centre emphasizes again the community and preventive aspects of medicine and in particular the organization and structure of health services. The basis of anesthetic practice, ophthalmology, and otorhinolaryngology is given during this year, using small group teaching and seminars. A course on medical ethics and forensic medicine is orientated specifically to local conditions.

During the last terms of the fourth year and the first two terms of the fifth year the students have a further ten-week clerkship in medicine and surgery and a five-week clerkship in pediatrics and obstetrics and gynecology. During these periods the student should be able to observe the entire pattern of medicine both in its curative and preventive aspects and the essential interrelationship of all disciplines. He also begins to assume more personal responsibility for patient care both in the wards and in the outpatient departments and clinics.

Examination and Assessment of Students

The progress of students throughout the course is measured first by assessment of their work in each subject during each term and second by university examinations that are held at the end of the first, second, and fifth years.

It is hoped that progressive assessment will allow a reduction in the magnitude of the final examinations.

APPENDIX 2

Regulations for the M.B., Ch.B. Degree at the University College, Dar Es Salaam

1. *Admission Requirements*: Candidates must satisfy the general entrance requirements of the University of East Africa. In addition candidates must offer passes in three of the following: physics, chemistry, and either biology or zoology. Of these at least one must be at the advanced level and the others at least at subsidiary standard of the Higher School Certificate or equivalent examination.

2. *Structure of the Curriculum*: The course of study extends over

five calendar years, including three academic years of a basic medical education program and two of clinical apprenticeships. In addition, students are required to complete satisfactorily a twelve-month internship.

3. *Details of the Curriculum*:

a) Basic Medical Education. This part of the course extends over a three-year period including nine terms of at least ten weeks' duration and two vacation terms of approximately six weeks each. The course includes basic scientific, clinical, and community aspects of medicine, correlated and partially integrated in each of the three years as follows:

First Year—Basic Biological Studies. The following topics/courses cover the subject of the healthy human being in his normal environment.

I. Cell and tissue biology—including an introduction to basic molecular biology and physicochemical aspects of tissue functions.

II. The natural history of the individual—including prenatal development (embryology), postnatal growth, development, and aging.

IV. The human body in health—correlative anatomy, physiology, and biochemistry of the major systems and regions of the body.

V. Human communities—social organization, introduction to human behavior, and factors affecting community health.

Second Year—Pathological Studies. The following topics/courses cover the subject of disease in the individual and the community.

I. General pathology—basic morphological and functional changes associated with disease processes in man.

II. Clinical laboratory procedures—including techniques used in the evaluation of patients and communities, especially microbiology, parasitology, and nutrition.

III. Social aspects of disease—including principles of epidemiology and statistics and their application to clinical and health problems in the family, small community, etc.

IV. The human being in disease—correlated/partially integrated morbid anatomy, pathological histology, and abnormal physiology/biochemistry of the major systems and regions of the body, and mental functions.

V. Clinical examination of patients—clinical observation including history-taking and physical examination of selected patients in order to illustrate abnormalities of the major systems, regions, and mental functions.

Third Year—Therapeutic Studies. The following topics/courses introduce the students to the management of disease in the individual and the community:

I. General pharmacology—principles of drug action in man, including metabolism and toxicology, and their effects on cells and tissues.

II. Applied pharmacology and therapeutics—including application of pharmacology to disease affecting the major systems, regions of the body, and mental functions.

III. Introduction to medical practice—participation in clinical work and instruction in the performance of common clinical procedures in medicine, surgery, and maternal and child care.

IV. Organization of medical care—including methods for control of community-wide endemic disease, promotion of health and care of handicapped persons, evaluation of therapeutic procedures applied to the community, and the organization of basic health services. Legal and ethical aspects of medical care.

V. Applied anatomy and physiology—a review of gross anatomy and clinical physiology applied to diagnosis and treatment.

b) Clinical Apprenticeships. During this phase of the course students are fully resident at a teaching hospital or its associated clinical units and health centers. They are regarded as junior members of the clinical and health teams to which they are assigned for intensive apprenticeships. They are not required to attend classes in the basic medical disciplines but are exposed to specially designed teaching activities in relation to clinical work, for example, clinical ward rounds, X-ray meetings, clinicopathological meetings, and therapeutic symposia.

Fourth Year—Junior Rotating Apprenticeships. The class is divided into six groups and rotated through the following postings: Two months each of medicine, surgery, pediatrics, obstetrics, health center practice, and special subjects. Fourth-year rotation occupies twelve months and the students are assigned specific tasks that they will hand over to their successors. Special subjects include medical and surgical assignments, particularly in psychiatry, venereology, ophthalmology, otology, radiology, and anesthesiology.

Fifth Year—Senior Rotating Apprenticeships. These last for eight months and the class is divided into four groups and rotated through the following: two months each of medicine, surgery, maternal and child health, and electives. Students carry out pathological procedures during their medical posting and give anesthetics during the surgical posting. During the elective period they are encouraged to participate in research programs, spend more time in a discipline of their choice or in a clinical apprenticeship in which their work has been unsatisfactory, or work in another faculty of medicine. In the last two months of the fifth year the entire class spends its time in reviewing and examinations.

APPENDIX 3
University of East Africa
Postgraduate Courses in the Faculty of Medicine

The provision of facilities for postgraduate training and education in the many disciplines of medicine is of the greatest importance. The medical journals bear witness to the numerous developments in the art and science of medicine that are taking place at such a pace that it is difficult for any one individual to be thoroughly conversant even with his own specialty and impossible for him to be familiar with every aspect of his profession.

Vocational training of medical practitioners in the environment in which they will work is of the utmost importance. Co-operation among the university faculties of medicine, the ministries of health and education, and the professional associations is obviously essential for the successful vocational training of medical practitioners.

Makerere University College medical school, in co-operation with the Ministry of Health, Uganda, has successfully carried out vocational training of medical graduates at Mulago Hospital for over twenty years. Hitherto the accent has been on preparing graduates for examinations organized by universities and professional colleges overseas. Such an arrangement is not conducive to the advancement of medicine in Africa and does not provide the solution to the high-level medical manpower requirements of East Africa in particular and Africa in general.

The third meeting of the East African Council for Medical Education was held on June 2, 1965, and after a full discussion between university and senior government officials from Uganda, Kenya, and Tanzania, agreement was reached on the following points:

1. That the establishment of East African postgraduate medical qualifications was highly desirable;
2. That the qualifications should be awarded by the University of East Africa;
3. That it would be desirable to aim at gaining international recognition for any East African qualifications instituted;
4. That it would be desirable to fully utilize all available training facilities in East Africa rather than send students overseas in large numbers for postgraduate training;
5. That the Board of the Faculty of Medicine should be requested to make specific recommendations to the Council on the courses of training that would be necessary, in order of priority, and on the control of standards of qualifications;
6. That the Board of the Faculty of Medicine be requested to make all necessary consultations with governments and local professional associations before making recommendations to the Council.

This statement was a landmark in the history of the development of postgraduate medical education in East Africa. The minutes stated in the clearest terms the philosophy behind the training programs leading to postgraduate medical qualifications to be awarded by the University of East Africa in its own right as a well-established institution for higher learning and research and as a member of the world community of universities.

The degrees of Master of Medicine (M.Med.) in medicine, surgery, obstetrics and gynecology, pediatrics, psychiatry, public health, and pathology, are designed as *specialist* professional qualifications at least equivalent to the postgraduate diplomas awarded by the royal colleges in Britain (M.R.C.P., M.R.C.O.G., F.R.C.S., etc.) or to the state specialty board certification in the United States

The standard of the diplomas in public health (D.P.H. [E.A.]), child health and tropical pediatrics (D.C.H. [E.A.]), and obstetrics (D.Obst. [E.A.]), will be equivalent to similar diplomas in Europe and North America.

Needless to say, the training programs for these postgraduate qualifications will be adapted to conditions and problems in Africa to a degree that could not possibly be achieved by postgraduate institutions in the developed countries. Steps will be taken however to enlist the co-operation or collaboration of postgraduate institutions overseas in the execution of these most significant training programs.

FREDERICK T. SAI
Head
Department of Preventive and Social Medicine
University of Ghana
Ghana Medical School
Accra, Ghana

WEST AFRICA

THE TOTAL POPULATION of West Africa's seventeen countries is probably around 220 million. According to United Nations' estimates, as of 1968, Nigeria, with an area of approximately 356,670 square miles, had a population of 62.6 million; Togo, with an area of 20,400 square miles, had 1.7 million; Ghana, with an area of 91,900 square miles had 8.3 million; and Gabon, which is about 9,000 square miles larger than Ghana, had 480,000. These are the orders of difference.

While some countries such as Ghana have accurate censuses, others have never attempted to take one. It is our hope that between 1970 and 1975 all West African countries will take some kind of census.

The division of the area into many small countries is one of the unfortunate obstacles to co-operative development. We should be developing regional schools, and yet our western neighbor, Ivory Coast, has an educational system that is sufficiently different from ours as to make this difficult. We have, however, established two associations in West Africa: the African Association of Surgeons, which is very effective but until recently lacked French-speaking representation, and the Association of Physicians which, although the weaker organization, does have reasonable French-speaking representation.

Before independence there was considerable co-operative effort between our medical field units and those of the French in the fight against endemic diseases and a great deal of interchange of information

---

Frederick Torgbor Sai received his M.B., B.S. from London University in 1953 and his B.Sc. in 1955. He had further training in tropical medicine and nutrition at the London School of Hygiene and Tropical Medicine and then took courses in internal medicine at Edinburgh University. He was elected to membership in the Royal College of Physicians in Edinburgh in 1959 and to fellowship in the college in 1964. He served in Ghana as a general duty medical officer specializing in human nutrition, and as a deputy chief medical officer. From 1963 to 1966 he was regional nutrition officer in Africa for the F.A.O. In 1966 he was appointed professor and head of the Department of Preventive and Social Medicine at the Ghana Medical School, a post he held until 1970 when he became director of medical services in Ghana.

and of supervisory personnel. This co-operation ceased with independence and the subsequent demographic changes that occurred in Africa. However, it now looks as though the stage is being set for a return to that kind of co-ordination and co-operation.

The differences in the economic levels of our respective countries and, therefore, in the priorities that they put on disease eradication and medical care in general, are also causes of major concern. Our northern neighbor, Upper Volta, is very poor compared to Ghana. Its government would balk at the kind of effort that we put into the control of, say, onchocerciasis. Yet without their joining in there is no point in starting a campaign for its eradication.

Certain facts about the population are of considerable importance to health and, incidentally, to medical education. One is that the growth rate of the West African population is between 2 and 3 per cent annually; the lowest rates are in the dry areas bordering the Sahara, where the people lead a nomadic life.

The over-all physician-population ratio is between 1:14,000 and 1:20,000. In some areas of Ghana it may range from 1:2,000 to 1:3,000, whereas, in areas such as Northern Nigeria it is between 1:150,000 and 1:200,000.

Health Problems

What then are the major health problems and the tasks to be performed?

At the top of the list I would put lack of information about health problems. Statistical information of any kind is completely lacking in most of the countries. In places where an effort has been made to collect data, the more they think they sharpen it the less accurate it becomes. For example, if someone states that there are a certain number of cases of diarrhea per 1,000 population it is more likely to be correct than if he states that there are a certain number of bacillary dysenteries per 1,000 population.

The direct governmental contribution to health care varies from about U.S. $1 to $3 per head. Consequently there is a lack of trained, qualified medical personnel and of health facilities of all kinds.

There is a shortage of national funds in general, not only funds for medical purposes. The unfortunate economic gap between African countries and Western countries seems to be widening at the same rate as the information gap is diminishing.

As for actual medical care problems, the demographic situation itself poses a serious question. The fertility rate (births per 1,000 people per year) ranges from 40:1,000 to 50:1,000. About 45 per cent of the population is under the age of fifteen years. Bringing children into the world, therefore, poses a major health challenge that we have to meet.

Life expectancy at birth is thirty-five to forty years; at age five it is fifty-five to fifty-eight years. This shows immediately the peculiar picture of life expectancy rising rather than falling from age zero to age six and demonstrates that health care for infants and preschool children presents a huge problem.

It is interesting to compare the rates of death at various ages. What are the causes of mortality and morbidity? In the first year there is what some describe as the respiratory-diarrhea complex, or pneumonia-diarrhea complex, where one is unable to ascribe any single etiological cause to the pneumonia or diarrhea that affects and kills so many children.

Then there are the infections in which the etiological agents are combined with malnutrition. Infections are responsible for 300 out of every 1,000 deaths, and that particular ratio is not declining significantly.

Another difficulty now confronting West Africans is the rapid rate of urbanization, which varies constantly from 7 to 10 to 12 per cent. This is several times the rate of demographic expansion and it is leading to urban conglomerates of various kinds that some of our colleagues have described as the "septic fringe," where people live and die in squalor, surrounded by disease.

Of the diseases presented at the health clinics and hospitals, in the more developed countries some 65 to 75 per cent are already under control or susceptible to simple treatment—diseases such as malaria, dysentery, and viral fevers of various kinds. In the urban areas, infectious hepatitis has become prevalent. Helminthic infections, enteric fevers, and, to a certain extent, tuberculosis and leprosy are still highly endemic diseases.

It is against this background that we see what is happening in the field of health care and what is likely to occur in the future.

A History of Medical Care in West Africa

Western medicine was introduced to West Africa by the Europeans, probably in the sixteenth century, and for a very long time it was restricted to Europeans and those with whom they were in immediate contact. Gradually it was extended to their servants and people working with them. It was not until after the smallpox campaigns had taken hold that medical care was expanded to cover the majority of the population, but then only under specific conditions that would help to safeguard the health of European residents.

After World War I it was recognized that some kind of expanded and more controlled medical care was necessary, and it was at this time that discussions began as to what kind of medical practitioner to train for West Africa.

The two principal external cultures to which West Africa had been exposed were the French and the British, and at the end of the war both countries established schools to train Africans to give medical care but not to be physicians.

The French called their program *Médecine Africaine,* training some students in Dakar and others in France. The British trainees were called "assistant medical officers" or "medical assistants" and received their training in Africa.

In concept this was not a bad idea; people were being trained locally to perform much-needed tasks. Where the project failed, or came up against a lot of subsequent opposition, was in the selection of the people to be trained and the length of training.

The best students available in any given year were selected and given three, four, and even five years of training in medicine and surgery, and then were permitted to work in the hospitals that were springing up in West Africa. What made the situation untenable was that both France and Britain were permissive enough to make it possible for other African students from affluent families to go to Europe for medical training.

The result was that some of the more intelligent but poor young men became assistant medical officers, while less bright ones went abroad and returned home as qualified physicians. In many instances those who had been trained locally under permanent supervision were, in a technical sense, more competent than the European graduates.

This situation quickly led to serious questioning of the validity of the local training programs, and in the end they were universally condemned and terminated.

What happened in the Congo is a classic example of how not to train medical personnel for Africa. In 1959–60 some Congolese assistant medical officers were sent to medical schools in France for training and became qualified physicians. But because of the sophisticated training they had received, when they returned it was found that they were not equipped to practice in the areas of West Africa where they were most needed.

At about this time the governments of West Africa began to accept total responsibility for the health care of their communities, although there was very little money and very few qualified personnel were available.

Current Trends in Medical Education

Although we condemned the old assistant medical officer system, all of us in West Africa have now moved toward an acceptance of the need for some kind of "doctor's extender" who can perform tasks for which the doctor has been overtrained.

In West Africa today both the French and British systems of medical education are followed. The oldest school in the French-speaking system is in Dakar, the other is in Abidjan. The schools in the English-speaking system are in Ibadan, Lagos, and Accra, while other schools are being developed in Zaria and in Monrovia. In Yaoundé, the capital of Cameroon, which is part French and part British, there is a French–British school.

It is my impression that the British system is currently more searching in its purposes and its adaptation to local conditions than is the French system. The latter will respond to change only if change takes place in France itself, whereas the British system constantly questions its role in Africa. The major difference between both the British and French local and metropolitan systems is that in the former greater emphasis is being placed on preventive and social medicine and on pediatrics and child health in general.

Rural Health Centers

In the field of preventive and social medicine the emphasis has taken the form of establishing demonstration areas. Each medical school is trying to develop a rural teaching center to which it can send its students to be trained. In order to ensure that the students will stay there, some of these centers are undergoing rapid changes in an effort to provide adequate living accommodations, teaching facilities, utilities, and other such necessities.

The Dakar medical school's demonstration area at Hombole is one of the more interesting, because it has a center for maternal and child health that has introduced a very important component—the rural midwifery practitioner. These rural midwives are brought into the demonstration area and taught elementary midwifery, including personal hygiene, the use of sterile equipment, and so forth. They are given presterilized packs to take out and, after delivering a child, they bring back the soiled pack, register the birth, and take out a new pack for the next delivery. The school has made good contact with the local community and its problems.

The demonstration center in Accra was established only recently. It covers a population of 25,000, a unit decided upon by the Ministry of Health, and was built with the help of the local people. It is hoped to demonstrate not only how to care for the health of the people but how to help them, through their leaders, to develop their own resources.

Within this context we hope to show that efficient, comprehensive community health care can be given at the outlay the government is prepared to spend, that is $2.50 per head.

Urban Health Centers

Most of our West African schools are failing to concentrate on the urban scene, which I think is a mistake because the cities are developing very rapidly. If we are to carry out experiments in extensive, comprehensive health care, the medical schools are going to have to develop urban counterparts to the rural health centers. This should be done not only at the undergraduate level but at the postgraduate, public-health training level also, because our municipalities are in a shocking state at the present time.

If it is our aim to develop residency programs for our physicians after they graduate, we must have good urban health establishments in which to place them. We have, therefore, made an arrangement with the officials of the municipality of Accra, which they welcome because they have been finding it difficult to get public health officers; the faculty of the Department of Preventive and Social Medicine of Ghana Medical School also act as assistant medical health officers in the city at the present time. We are trying to get the city's organization running smoothly so that we can feed our students into it when they reach the second year of their two-year post-qualifying program, which starts after the preregistration year.

Training the Health Team

Another major problem area is how to integrate the training of the health team at certain points and how to encourage members of the team to relate to one another when working in the field. This is not an easy task because of the dichotomy in their training. Throughout West

Africa the medical student is trained along traditional lines within the medical school; all other health personnel are trained in schools operated by the ministries of health. The relationship between the ministries, the other units of the universities, and the medical schools is far from cordial, especially in the English-speaking countries. The ministries have an "anti-bright boy" complex, while the universities think the medical schools get too much money and "seduce" too many students away from the university in general. In many countries this situation has made it impossible for these groups to sit down and talk together.

An experiment that has been started at Ibadan seems to hold out hope. With the support of the World Health Organization and The Rockefeller Foundation the university has set up a graduate nurses' program in which they are enrolling some nurses for degree courses and upgrading the training of others. The program is in very close relationship to the medical school.

Ibadan is also trying to establish a medical science degree for sanitarians in an endeavor to narrow the gap that exists between these important health workers and the physicians. It is hoped that this training will, within reasonable limits, enable the sanitarians to communicate with the physicians about their subject.

Training the Nurse

Another primary target is nursing education. After receiving the high school diploma a would-be registered nurse is given three years' training. In some areas a qualified nurse has had only ten years of formal education before taking the course. The nurse-midwife and the midwife also have had ten years of schooling followed by two years of training.

Under the British system the public health nurse, or health visitor, has three years of nurses' training, one year of midwifery training, and one year of public health nurses' training. Much of this lengthy training is superfluous, but it does go into the making of a professional as opposed to an auxiliary—the community health nurse who trains for only two years after ten years of formal education.

Under the French system the levels are comparable although not exactly alike. For example, the *Infirmiere Sociale* is not identical to our public health nurse; the former is also something of a community development officer—more of a combination nurse and social welfare worker.

TRAINING THE MEDICAL AUXILIARY

There are, therefore, two completely different grades to consider: the professional and, at all levels, the auxiliary. If our health educators would look at the situation that way, we would have a professional training program for physicians, nurses, and other paramedical personnel, and a training program for auxiliaries. We are recruiting our physicians' auxiliaries from among nurses. We have two types of auxiliaries to the public health nurse and the nurse-midwife: the midwife and the community health nurse.

Eventually we hope that the demonstration areas will be under the control of a council on medical education. In the meantime, we are trying to set up an orientation or workshop practice group that will include newly qualified physicians, medical students, other professional paramedical workers, and auxiliaries, and place them as a team in the rural areas. Seminars will be held before they go, or in the evenings, and we will attempt to map out for them clearly what each may and may not do. If we take this approach I foresee that the physician will know the extent to which he can depend on the medical auxiliary, the public health nurse, and the other personnel.

It will be necessary to organize the health services in such a way that everyone knows precisely the level at which the auxiliaries can perform and the amount of supervision they require.

Every unit of 25,000 population should have one physician's auxiliary at the head of its health care center. Working under him would be two midwives, a community health nurse, and an auxiliary sanitarian. The most peripherally situated health team would consist of auxiliaries only, headed by an auxiliary physician and supervised by a qualified physician who would be in a position to assess their work and give them continual guidance.

Once a year or so these auxiliaries should be brought back to a regional orientation center for reassessment; there is nothing more demoralizing to these people than to leave them on their own year after year with no opportunity to learn about new developments that are taking place.

The difficulty with the old auxiliary physician system, as I mentioned earlier, was that they were selected from a group that could have qualified for medical school and then given training that was close to but not quite on the level of a physician's training. We are advocating that in choosing those to be trained as physicians' auxiliaries we should be quite sure that they are under no circumstances qualified to enter medical school, and that they be trained for very specifically oriented tasks that they will perform later. They should be supervised in such a way that they will not consider themselves as physicians. We feel that this may be a more constructive approach.

In West Africa a major challenge is how to look at the medical tasks to be performed, the health services that exist, and the funds available, and devise training programs that will make it possible to bring everyone into contact with health services at all times.

Health Center Superintendents

Up until recently, immediately after graduation, health center superintendents were assigned to hospitals where they screened patients under the supervision of a doctor. When they were judged competent to tell which patients they could treat and which should be referred to a doctor they were sent out to supervise a health center.

The training of superintendents started in about 1950 and continued until 1963, when the government decided that we had sufficient doctors to man all the health centers and that the training of superintendents should be stopped. The training was curtailed and the doctors came to the centers but, in terms of the problems to be faced, they were not as capable as the superintendents. As a result of this situation, we had on our hands a fine corps of trained men who were unhappy, and a group of doctors who had been brought in to do a task for which they had not been trained who were also unhappy.

It took until 1968 for this situation to change and for the project to be re-established. Two of us were charged with the responsibility of working up the details of the training and functions of the superintendents. The training has now started; we are still working on the functions.

Under the present system, a health center superintendent must be a male who has had ten to twelve years of formal education, completed a three to four-year nursing course, and acquired a qualified registered nurse's diploma. He must also have practiced satisfactorily as a nurse for ten years.

After passing an entrance examination he enters a one-year training course in which he is taught to diagnose and treat elementary diseases and to administer a health center.

After training they will probably be placed in a smaller unit than a health center, which is supposed to serve a population of 100,000. The proper place for the superintendents is in a unit serving 25,000 people, where they will be in over-all charge. They will do mostly clinical work and will be responsible for the community health nurses, who are really the health educators of the community. An auxiliary sanitarian will be based at the unit, also, to do the environmental work in the community.

For a country in need of paramedical personnel we think this is a good system. In Ghana, for example, the nurses were beginning to be dissatisfied because of the lack of opportunities for promotion and similar factors. Giving them this further training as an avenue of promotion is good for them and good for the country.

I believe that in the future, medical education in West Africa will move more in the direction of the doctor being a "managerial physician." He will have to know how to operate and monitor equipment that will do various laboratory tests and techniques and provide results quickly. In addition he will have to know how to deploy and supervise paramedical personnel so that they will have more responsibility for patient care. We will have fewer doctors, a great many more auxiliaries, and very sophisticated medical equipment. I think this is the sensible direction for future developments to take.

Health Education

When we were children, as part of a general over-all attack on diseases such as malaria, practical health education was taught in almost all schools. When DDT and penicillin were introduced such instruction ceased, due to a comfortable feeling that it was no longer necessary. We had the means to attack disease so people thought they no longer had to teach health education.

We are now swinging away from that attitude. A health education unit has been created in the Ministry of Health, which is now consulting with the Ministry of Education to try to find out how health education may be introduced.

Family planning has now been accepted as a national policy, so we are going to have a transfusion into the program. We maintain that education in family planning should incorporate education for the general improvement of maternal and child health care.

It would be interesting to try to develop primary health care education centers in relation to the school system, but I see difficulties immediately in such countries as Tanzania and Uganda. In parts of Uganda, for example, villages as we understand them do not exist and the population is so scattered that a child might be quite a distance away from a school. Even in Ghana some of the schools are a long way from the villages they serve. It might be possible, however, to introduce such centers in the larger villages.

JOSÉ CUYEGKENG
Executive Director
Association of Philippine Medical Colleges
Manila, The Philippines

THE PHILIPPINES

THE PRESENT Republic of the Philippines is the third in our history, the first having been established during the revolution against the Spaniards in 1898. It ended with the American occupation in 1900. The second republic was established by the Japanese armed forces in 1943 and was also short-lived, ending with the liberation of the islands by the Allies in 1945. The third republic was founded in 1946 when independence was granted by the United States.

The Philippines is an archipelago consisting of about 7,000 islands of which only about 20 to 30 are inhabited to an appreciable degree. Based on the 1960 census it has a projected estimated population of 38 million at the present time, with a growth rate of 3.2 to 3.5 per cent a year. The population is very young: 45 per cent is under the age of fifteen.

If a literate person is defined as one who has finished at least four years of elementary education, the literacy rate in the Philippines is between 75 and 80 per cent. Whether these people are able to read and write adequately, however, I do not know.

There are an estimated 15,000 physicians in the country today and another 9,000 in other countries, 95 per cent of whom are in the United States. Approximately 6,000 of these are permanent residents of the United States who are practicing medicine; about 3,000 are in hospital internships and residencies.

THE HISTORY OF MEDICAL EDUCATION

With this background let me briefly describe the history of medical education in the Philippines.

José Cuyegkeng received his M.D. degree from the University of the Philippines in 1945 and his M.P.H. degree from the University of Michigan School of Public Health in 1951. He was a member of the faculty of the University of the Philippines College of Medicine from 1946 to 1956. In 1956 he became professor of pathology and microbiology and head of the department at the University of the East College of Medicine, Ramon Magsaysay Memorial Medical Center. He was dean of the College of Medicine from 1963 to 1969, when he was appointed executive director of the Association of Philippine Medical Colleges.

Formal higher education started with the authorization from Rome to establish the Royal Pontifical University of Santo Tomas, which was founded in 1611; authorization for a medical faculty was not given until 1871. The first students admitted to the medical school were those who had finished a "bacheller," the equivalent of the present-day high school diploma.

Until 1907 the medical curriculum was of three years' duration, with one year preclinical and two years' clinical, leading to a licentiate in medicine.

Following the American occupation in 1900, the Governor General authorized a second medical school which began operation in 1907 and became a unit of the University of the Philippines in 1908. Again, requirement for admission was the equivalent of a high school diploma. The medical course was extended to four years—two preclinical and two clinical—and an internship of one year was required before the medical degree was granted.

It was not until 1935 that a third medical school was founded; it was the first proprietary medical school to be established.

Until the outbreak of World War II the three schools admitted between 300 and 500 freshman students annually and had an output of about 300 graduates a year.

During the Japanese occupation the University of the Philippines medical school was the only institution of higher learning allowed to continue in operation. Teaching at the University of Santo Tomas medical school was curtailed for a year because its teaching hospital and school building had been demolished during the battles to liberate Manila. The private medical school remained closed during the occupation.

The only important change to take place between 1907 and 1945 was that medical school admission requirements increased to two years of college; a student needed a total of seventy-two credits in a college of arts and sciences. Thus the educational requirement to enter medical school consisted roughly of seven years of primary education, four years of secondary education, and two years of college.

The end of the war brought with it a strong demand by students for higher education. A great backlog of those in the student age group wanted to attend a university. Since the government was bankrupt at that time, the only way to satisfy this demand was for private individuals to try to find the capital to open colleges and even universities.

In 1947 the old private medical school was reactivated, and between that year and 1957 four more private schools were established. Today we have seven medical schools, one government-supported (University of the Philippines), one run by a religious order (University of Santo Tomas), and five run by private sources. Of the latter, only one is operated on a nonprofit basis.

Because of the large number of students who wanted to study medicine, and because of the attraction that upon graduation they would be eligible to enter the United States under the Exchange Visitors' Program, medical school freshman admissions in the 1950's ranged from a low of 100 in the state-supported school to a high of 1,200 in one of the private schools. Total freshman enrollment in the seven schools was from 3,000 to 4,000 students in a given year.

At the end of the first year the dropout rate was very high—from 30 to 50 per cent. Of those who survived the first year, less than 30 per cent would graduate on schedule; some would require from six to eight years to finish the course. During the 1950's there was an annual output of about 2,000 physicians, or about 50 per cent of those who had entered medical school.

Curtailing Enrollment

In 1957–58 the former dean of the University of the Philippines made a study to determine how many students should be enrolled in the medical school in order for the income from their tuition to support the school adequately. The subsequent estimate was that total enrollment should not be less than 1,200.

By 1960 it became obvious that we were admitting too many students to medical school and that the dropout rate was extremely high. In co-operation with the Philippine Mission of the United States Agency for International Development and the Council of Deans, it was agreed to place a limitation on medical school enrollment. Under the leadership of Dr. Lloyd Florio, and with A.I.D. support, a project was launched to make available twelve two-year fellowships a year for four years in the basic sciences, and $1 million for the purchase of equipment and supplies for the teaching faculties of the seven medical schools.

One condition for the schools' participation in this program was the voluntary reduction in freshman enrollment. The result was that over a period of four years, a school admitting 1,200 freshmen would reduce this number to no more than 300. For the past two years, total freshman enrollment in the seven medical schools has ranged from 1,400 to 1,600 students.

The Medical Act

Medical education in the Philippines is under the control of the Board of Medical Education whose decisions take precedence over those of the Department of Education. The board is authorized by the Medical Act of 1959 to impose the requirements for admission to medical school.

The act stated the admissions requirements as follows: Beginning in 1963 a baccalaureate degree would be required, meaning that a student must have completed seven years of elementary education, four years of high school, and four years of college. The act specified the courses that must be taken and the number of units needed to obtain the baccalaureate degree, so that the degree would not be an end course in itself. Students who finished the course and failed to enter medical school would be a liability to the community, so in order to qualify to teach, say, natural science or biology in high school or college, they would have to go through another year of college and earn a second baccalaureate degree.

Selection

Each medical school, especially the University of Santo Tomas, has a well-organized system for selecting students for admission. In January and February they give examinations in various regions of the archipelago. After this preliminary screening they request the students to submit their academic records for further screening. The third step is for a panel of faculty members to interview prospective students in order to decide on who should be admitted.

Three years ago the Board of Medical Education decided that all applicants to medical school must take a medical college admissions test. The test is being prepared by the Philippine Psychological Association. At present no definite passing mark in this test has been made. The question of how the results of the test are to be correlated with the students' performance in medical school is still being studied.

Medical Curriculum

There have been very few changes in the medical curriculum: it still consists of two years' preclinical, two years' clinical, and a one-year rotating internship. Individual schools have modified the curriculum by adding new subjects such as medical psychology, by introducing more courses in preventive and social medicine, and by reducing the number of course hours, especially in anatomy. During the past few years all the schools have displayed a greater interest in incorporating courses on community medicine into the curriculum.

Two years ago, medical school faculty members stated that they wished to review the curriculum. So, prior to the first National Conference on Medical Education in May 1968, we held a series of preconference seminars as a result of which definite steps are being taken to make desirable changes in the medical school curriculum. In order to do this it was necessary to modify the existing Medical Act. This was accomplished during the last session of Congress in June of this year.

Realizing that the premedical curriculum as specified in the act is too rigid, we were able to convince Congress to amend this section so that the subjects and number of units to be taken for a baccalaureate degree are not specified and the degree will be an end course in itself.

Under the amendment to the act, whereby a baccalaureate degree is the only requirement needed to qualify for entrance to medical school, it is believed that the Board of Medical Education will impose certain other requirements, such as that students who want to take up medicine as a career will probably need to major in the natural or biological sciences. Apart from that, the number of units or subjects to be taken will not be specified.

Under the amendment, also, an eight-member Board of Medical Education has been set up, chaired by the Secretary of Education. The other members include the Secretary of Health, the Director of the Bureau of Private Schools, the Chairman of the Board of Medical Examiners, the Dean of the College of Medicine of the University of the Philippines, and representatives of the Philippine Medical Association (P.M.A.), the Association of Philippine Medical Colleges (A.P.M.C.), and the Council of Deans of Philippine Medical Schools.

At present the medical degree is given after the one-year rotating internship. In the future the degree may be given after the fourth year of medical school, although one year of internship, the nature of which has yet to be determined by the board, will still be a requirement for the licensing examination. We are looking forward to the time when the rotating internship will be replaced by either a straight or a mixed internship.

This change will allow the implementation of some of the conclusions arrived at in the preconference seminars and at the conference itself, when a great majority of faculty members stated that the four-year course could well be given in three years and that the fourth year could be a one-year internship within the medical school. They believe that the additional one-year internship outside of the university was, in a way, meant to solve the problem of not having enough physicians to staff our peripheral hospitals.

Health Care in the Rural Areas

We believe that if we cannot control the flow of our graduates to the United States, we can at least require that they serve the country in the peripheral hospitals for one year before they go abroad.

This step was taken as a compromise with Congress, because every year for the past ten years some congressman or senator has wanted to file a bill requiring that all graduates serve in a rural area for two years.

The P.M.A. and the A.P.M.C. have always taken a firm stand against such legislation, stating to the Congress that unless and until there are adequate logistics to support the graduates while they practice in the rural areas it is a waste of their time to go there.

In response to the need for health care in the rural areas, for the past three years each of the seven medical schools has established so-called comprehensive community medicine demonstration areas in rural communities. The students are exposed to these programs in their third and fourth years, and spend some time working on them during their internships.

The Private Schools

Ninety-two per cent of the physician population are graduates of the private medical schools. Because of the voluntary reduction in enrollment in the five schools and, at the same time, the improvement in facilities and the increase in faculty size, they are now reaching the point where they may have to close because of financial difficulties.

Three years ago the deans and administrators of these schools agreed that as of January 1970 they would change their corporate structure and begin to operate on a nonstock, nonprofit basis, which will probably enable them to put sufficient pressure on the government to subsidize them. Actually, in 1965 Congress did authorize such subsidies to the private schools, in view of the fact that they had to maintain teaching hospitals with a minimum of 100 free beds. Once all of these schools are on a nonprofit basis, however, we will be in a stronger position to get them the necessary support from the government.

Licensing

With the improved communication between the medical schools and the drastic cut in freshman enrollment, the performance of the graduates in the state licensing examination has improved considerably. Two examinations are given each year and in the past four examinations only 10 to 15 per cent failed. On a national basis the poorer schools have made definite improvements.

Some faculty members in the three nonprofit schools assist in the teaching at the four profit-making schools. When I was dean of the medical faculty of the University of the East, however, we made it a policy that none of our faculty members could teach at another medical school. This was not because we wanted to limit their activities but because most of them taught on a part-time basis and I could not see how they could do so in another school as well and still maintain a private practice.

Through the A.P.M.C. we have broken down the barriers between the medical schools, and, indeed, one of the programs we hope the University of the Philippines will agree to undertake is to send visiting professors to other medical schools and thus bring about an improvement in instruction in the poorer schools.

Postgraduate Training

We still face great problems at the undergraduate educational level, but we hope in the next decade to reduce the length of the premedical course, as well as the medical course itself, in the belief that there is a great need for our graduates to receive postgraduate training.

We are so much involved with improving our undergraduate programs that the only postgraduate program we have is for residents, the nature of which is more or less dictated by the specialty societies. Residency training is four years for medicine, five for surgery, three for pediatrics, and three for obstetrics and gynecology.

The specialty societies have begun to organize boards that will give examinations to those who wish to qualify as specialists. The Civil Service Commission has recognized the specialty boards and once a physician has been certified by one of them the government will automatically consider him a qualified specialist.

Almost all continuing education is supervised by the P.M.A. in co-operation with the faculties of the seven medical schools. We feel that the schools should take an active part in such programs, but because of problems peculiar to our country it is doubtful that they will be able to do so for the next few years.

The Exodus of Medical Personnel

A review of the activities of the graduates of all seven medical schools over the past several years shows that as many as 80 per cent do not go into practice after licensure. Instead they seek residency training in teaching hospitals. But the hospitals can absorb no more than 20 per cent of the graduates, and that is the reason they go to the United States.

It is a curious phenomenon that instead of attempting to increase our production of physicians we have undertaken a course to reduce the output because of a disequilibrium in the economy that results in our being unable to support a greater number of physicians. It is not that the funds are not available; it is simply a matter of the government giving a very low priority to the delivery of health services.

Although many of our graduates know full well that some of the hospitals in the United States to which they will be appointed have no valid training programs, they still go there in order to earn money. Eventually many of them seek permanent residence in the United States and continue to staff community hospitals as house physicians because of their inability to earn a living in the Philippines.

Under an arrangement with the Educational Council for Foreign Medical Graduates in the United States, it will not certify a Philippine medical graduate who has passed the E.C.F.M.G. examination unless he is registered to practice in the Philippines.

Paramedical personnel are also leaving the country for the same reason—the economy cannot support them. There are, for example, about 12,000 Philippine nurses in the United States.

The problem has been under discussion for the past few years. Some people see the exodus as beneficial, because if we were to prevent these people from leaving, as was done in India, we would have a very serious unemployment problem. At the same time, economists feel that not only are these people serving humanity, albeit not in their own country, but they are increasing the dollar income of the Philippines, since most of them send money home to help support their families. Others feel that a great deal of time and money has been spent to produce these physicians and paramedical personnel and that this has not been a good investment.

The Future of Medical Care

It is our hope that a concerted effort by the P.M.A. and the A.P.M.C. will convince the government to give a higher priority to the appropriation of funds for the delivery of health services. If rapport can be established between the medical schools and the departments of health and education, eventually the schools will play a major role in formulating health programs for the country.

It is unfortunate that this is an election year. Special health funds were to have been provided by a health tax, but this measure did not go through the Senate because it had already passed several unpopular tax bills. But to demonstrate that the communication gap between the professionals and the politicians is narrowing, the Congress did pass a special science tax that will generate about 50 million pesos a year to support science in general. It also passed a special education measure that will bring in about 150 million pesos.

This means that real estate taxes will be increased. They have been 1½ per cent but an additional 1 per cent has been added that will be earmarked specifically for general education. This is in addition to the regular appropriation in the education budget.

This year, under the auspices of the P.M.A., Congress approved a medical care program. We are well aware that to embark on a nation-wide program of health care would bring the government to bankruptcy. Due to the insistence of the A.P.M.C. and other organizations the government has agreed to make a two-year study of the problems. The measure is known as the Medicare Act and its objective is the delivery of medical services; the first step was to create a Medical Care Commission. Under the act, the commission has been given two years to draw up and submit to Congress a list of recommendations as to how this objective can be achieved.

SJAHRIAR RASAD
Dean
University of Indonesia
Faculty of Medicine
Djakarta, Indonesia

INDONESIA

INDONESIA IS an archipelago near the equator consisting of more than 3,000 islands the largest of which are Borneo, Sumatra, Celebes, and Java. The greatest distance between the eastern and western borders of the archipelago is about 3,500 miles. The total population as of 1968 was 112.8 million of which perhaps 80 million live on Java, the smallest of the four larger islands, which makes Java the most densely populated area in the world with 1,000 people per square mile.

While the soil is very rich the people are very poor. The per capita income is estimated roughly at U.S. $80 a year, probably one of the lowest figures in the world.

Ninety per cent of the people are Muslims, about 8 per cent are Christians, and the rest are Buddhists or Hindus. The population is composed of heterogeneous ethnic groups who speak different dialects, but one standard language—Bahasa Indonesia—is understood and spoken by all groups. Bahasa Indonesia is the medium of instruction at all levels of education.

THE DEVELOPMENT OF MEDICAL EDUCATION

It may be instructive to trace the various stages of development of medical education in Indonesia in order to understand many of the problems inherent in contemporary medical education in this country of ethnically heterogeneous people. Medical education has always been

Sjahriar Rasad obtained his M.D. from the University of Indonesia Faculty of Medicine in 1945. He took postgraduate training in radiology in London, Stockholm, Paris, and New York and was certified by the American Board of Radiology in 1950. In 1957 he was appointed professor of radiology and head of the department at the University of Indonesia medical school, a position he now holds. He was elected dean of the Faculty of Medicine in 1964 and remained in that post until 1970. In 1967 he was elected an honorary fellow of the American College of Radiology. Currently he is a member of the Consortium of Medical Sciences, a national board that supervises medical education in Indonesia, and, as his country's representative, a member of the Central Coordinating Board of Tropical Medicine and Public Health of the South East Asian Ministers of Education Organization.

closely linked with the development of Indonesian society as a whole. The first medical training program was established more than a century ago in a colonial environment and therefore manifested a number of patterns inevitably associated with colonial society. The present structure of medical education in Indonesia is much more in accordance with the nature of a free modern society.

In the middle of the nineteenth century the island of Java was virtually under the control of the Dutch colonial government which had its seat in Batavia, now called Djakarta. I should emphasize that when I say "colonial government" I mean the prewar Dutch government; by no means do I refer to the present Dutch government, for relations between the people and governments of our two countries are very good at the present time.

At that time the Dutch launched smallpox eradication campaigns and a number of Javanese vaccinators, the indigenous inhabitants of Central and East Java, were the first native individuals to acquire a knowledge of modern medicine. In order to formalize training in smallpox vaccination, in 1851 the Dutch established a small school for the training of native medical practitioners.

The school was attached to the Military Hospital in Batavia and started with only thirteen students, who were expected to study for one year. The teaching staff consisted of Dutch military physicians who taught in the Malay language which, while known in the archipelago, was not the native tongue of the indigenous inhabitants of Java. Medical terms were taught in their Latin form.

It was soon recognized that the students could also be trained to diagnose common diseases, perform minor surgery, and treat some illnesses, so the duration of study was immediately extended to two years. At the end of this period the students were examined by a commission of Dutch military physicians and pharmacists and those who passed were granted the title of *dokter Djawa,* or Javanese physician.

In 1875 the medical training program was extended to five or six years with instruction in Dutch; a preparatory course was included in the program to enable the candidates to learn Dutch. Later, new students were recruited from among the native graduates of the so-called European elementary schools where the language of instruction was Dutch. This program not only produced the first native medical practitioners but also the first nationalist leaders such as Abdul Rivai and Radjiman Wediodiningrat.

In 1902 a new development occurred with the transfer of the old *dokter Djawa* school from the Military Hospital to its own building, complete with residential quarters for 200 students. The school was reorganized and renamed the School tot Opleinding van Inlandsche Artsen (S.T.O.V.I.A.), or the School for the Training of Native Physicians. The term "inlandsche artsen," native physician, was changed in 1913 to "Indische artsen," Indian physician. S.T.O.V.I.A. had two divisions: a preparatory three-year program characteristic of a junior high school program, and a seven-year medical program.

The students, until 1913 exclusively natives, were usually recruited from the Dutch-language elementary schools. First-division students were given scholarships; financial support was given to those in the second division who requested it. After graduation those on scholarships were expected to serve the colonial government as medical practitioners for eight years and were assigned to various places in the archipelago.

Two years after the school was put into operation a change in the Higher Education Law in Holland gave graduates of S.T.O.V.I.A. the right to take the theoretical medical examinations given by the medical faculties in Holland. This meant that S.T.O.V.I.A. graduates did not have to take the so-called candidate or first-degree examination in order to continue their medical training and earn a physician's diploma from a Dutch medical school, and quite a number of them took advantage of this opportunity.

In 1913 the colonial government established a second medical school, the Nederlandsch-Indische Artsen School (N.I.A.S.), or the Netherlands-Indies School of Physicians. In contrast to S.T.O.V.I.A., N.I.A.S. was not exclusively for native students; it also enrolled a few of European and Chinese descent.

Located in Surabaja in East Java, the school's educational program was the same as that of S.T.O.V.I.A. in Batavia. It had excellently equipped laboratories and, for clinical training, a large hospital with dispensaries and clinics.

In both schools emphasis was placed upon the practical aspects of medicine rather than upon its purely scientific aspects, and graduates were fully qualified to practice medicine, surgery, and obstetrics in the colony but not in Holland.

In 1920 the first institution of higher education was established—a technical college in Bandung financed by private Dutch and business interests. Seven years later the Dutch established a medical college in Batavia. It opened with a staff of professors of anatomy, physiology, pathology and pathological anatomy, surgery, and internal diseases. The first class consisted of 24 students in contrast to the 160 who were studying at S.T.O.V.I.A. By the 1934–35 academic year 471 students were enrolled: 88 Europeans, 158 Chinese, and 225 native Indonesians. They were recruited from the graduate body of the five-year Dutch high school, known as H.B.S., or from schools that issued the equivalent of an H.B.S. diploma.

Under a law passed in December 1934 the diploma of the medical college in Batavia was held to be equal to those granted by faculties of medicine in Holland. Moreover, transfer to a Dutch university would no longer involve the repetition of examinations in subjects already passed successfully in Batavia.

The study program at the college was divided into three parts, concluding with the candidate, doctoral, and arts examinations. A student was expected to take the first part of the candidate examination at the end of his first year and the second part two years later. The doctoral examination was normally scheduled for the end of the fifth year, but much depended on the faculty who determined the required period of study for each individual student. Only after a student had passed the doctoral examination was he entitled to take the arts examination. Upon passing it he was granted the diploma of arts.

The medical college was closed in 1942 when the Japanese armed forces attacked the colony and forced the Dutch to surrender. The Japanese occupational government soon acknowledged the necessity for the continuation of medical training, however, and the medical college in Batavia was opened in 1943 with the Japanese name, Ika Daigaku, or Medical Faculty.

Since the Dutch members of the prewar teaching staff were in concentration camps, a fate shared by all who could not claim to be of Indonesian descent, native physicians were appointed to the staff to work with Japanese professors in providing medical instruction.

The prohibition against using the Dutch language, regarded by the Japanese as the language of the enemy, compelled the Indonesian faculty members to teach in their own language and to create in a very short time a modern medical vocabulary in the Indonesian language. A special commission created a basic Indonesian scientific vocabulary and it was put to use immediately. Thus developed the basis for the emergence of a new national language that is also suitable for scientific discourse.

On August 17, 1945, in behalf of the Indonesian people, Sukarno and Muhammad Hatta proclaimed the independence of Indonesia. Students at the medical college in Djakarta, formerly Batavia, took an active part in the preparations for this historical event. (The ensuing events, with Japanese military personnel still in power and Allied troops coming in, did not permit any orderly resumption of educational activities.)

The return of the Dutch colonial government forced the supporters of the newly established republic to defend their freedom. Many faculty members and students followed the Indonesian Republican government in its retreat to the interior of Central Java where they established their stronghold in Djokjakarta.

There medical education was soon reorganized and courses began, although under very difficult circumstances. Owing to the lack of adequate facilities classes were scattered over more than one town. Teachers and students frequently had to leave to fight the invading Dutch military forces. In this revolutionary environment it was only natural that instruction was often given in the Indonesian language.

In 1948 the scattered educational units were brought together to constitute the Faculty of Medicine of the newly established University of Gadjah Mada in Djokjakarta.

Upon its return to Indonesia immediately after the war, the Dutch colonial government had established a temporary university in Djakarta which in 1947 was named the University of Indonesia. When the Indonesian Republican government finally succeeded in returning to Djakarta in the beginning of 1950 the university was virtually a Dutch institution.

Because so many Indonesians were in the interior fighting the Dutch, very few native students had been re-enrolled. In the first academic year there had been 103 Dutch and 98 Chinese students, but only 9 Indonesians. In 1948, 251 students were enrolled. In the same year the Faculty of Medicine at Surabaja, established by the returning Dutch on the foundations of the old N.I.A.S., had only 37 students. Almost all the faculty members in both institutions were Dutch, and instruction was given in that language. Gradually the Dutch teachers were replaced by Indonesians and eventually all instruction was given in Indonesian. Foreign professors were, however, permitted to teach in English.

The transition from a Dutch faculty, rooted in the Western European academic tradition, to an Indonesian faculty more receptive to deviations from established academic patterns, was facilitated by the generous co-operation extended by the University of California. In 1954 the government of the United States made it possible for the faculty to establish an affiliation with the University of California that facilitated the training of faculty for undergraduate and graduate teaching and the acquisition of basic equipment necessary for the implementation of modern medical training.

By 1955 the old seven-year curriculum inherited from the prewar medical college was no longer considered satisfactory. A new six-year system of supervised study was introduced to conform to modern concepts of medical education and to the urgently felt needs of the Indonesian people.

In the ensuing six years 26 American visiting professors taught at the Faculty of Medicine of the University of Indonesia, thus assisting in its initial development as a modern medical school. In addition 6 technical experts contributed their share as visiting instructors. More than 100 Indonesian physicians and other experts, both senior and junior members of the teaching staff, received fellowships to do advanced work in the United States and in other countries for periods ranging from three months to three years.

The China Medical Board of New York rendered assistance in various forms and played an active role in setting up the affiliation program with the University of California. The board continues to support the medical faculty with annual grants for the purchase of laboratory equipment, books and journals for the library, and two fellowships each year. A special grant from the board made it possible to establish a new Department of Parasitology. In 1960 the affiliation with the University of California was terminated and there was mutual agreement that it had been a most satisfactory relationship.

Additional Medical Faculties

Following international recognition of the Republic of Indonesia in 1949, the government, mindful of the increasing demands of the people for better living conditions, including accessibility to medical care, began to establish additional medical faculties. Until that time medical faculties existed only at the University of Indonesia in Djakarta, Gadjah Mada University in Djokjakarta, and Airlangga University in Surabaja. Subsequently, medical faculties were founded at the following universities:

1955: University of North Sumatra in Medan on Sumatra
University of Hasanuddin in Macassar on Celebes
1957: University of Andalas in Padang on Sumatra
University of Padjadjaran in Bandung on Java

More recently additional faculties have been established and we now have a total of eleven government-operated facilities; the newer ones are:

Sam Ratulangi University in Manado on Celebes
Diponegoor University in Semarang on Java
University of Sriwidjaja in Palembang on Sumatra
University of Udayana in Denpasar on Bali

There are also a number of private medical schools, most of them in Djakarta, only a few of which have their own hospitals and laboratories. There is really no reason for the existence of these schools and they present our biggest problem. Many were founded by adventurers, under the law of higher education that permits any academician to start a university. They have no curriculum worth mentioning.

As an example, the so-called Santa Paula University was established three years ago in a small room of a church. They try to attract our faculty members to lecture and because our staff are so underpaid by the government most of them accept these invitations in order to increase their incomes.

The rapid expansion of new medical faculties all over the archipelago inevitably led to the necessity of making plans to ensure that the new schools will not be forced to lower their academic standards because of lack of adequate facilities.

Accordingly, in 1962 the government designated the Faculty of Medicine of the University of Indonesia to act as a "feeder" to the other faculties and gave it the responsibility for:

1. Training the teaching staff of the newer faculties;
2. Providing educational facilities (clerkships, internships, etc.) for students from these faculties in specialties not adequately available in their own schools; and
3. Providing teaching staff and technical assistance to the other faculties on either a temporary or permanent basis.

Training of the Faculty

When it was founded in 1927 the present Faculty of Medicine of the University of Indonesia had a teaching staff of 6 professors and 7 extraordinary professors. The present staff consists of 620 physicians: 40 full professors, 50 assistants professors, 93 lecturers, 21 junior lecturers, and 316 assistants.

The number of specialized departments has also increased, and almost all of them are headed by a full professor; only in exceptional cases, mostly in the preclinical fields, are the departments headed by assistant professors.

Almost all professors, assistant professors, and lecturers have had specialized training abroad, particularly in the United States, Canada, the United Kingdom, and the Netherlands. Many are fully certified by foreign specialty boards, such as the American Board of Radiology, the British Pediatric Society, and the Dutch Society of Surgeons. Over the past decade more than 100 members of the teaching staff participated in international conferences and contributed to foreign journals.

The University Hospital in Djakarta, with 1,500 beds, is the largest in the country and is equipped with modern technical facilities. For example, the Department of Radiology is fully equipped to do radiodiagnostic and therapeutic procedures, including angiography and cesium and cobalt therapy.

Curriculum

The six-year study program is divided into three parts: one year of premedical, two years of preclinical, and three years of clinical training. The first three years are each divided into semesters. Junior clerkship begins in the fourth year and senior clerkship is done in the fifth and sixth years.

The curriculum is organized as follows:

First year: Biology, chemistry, and physics.

Second year: Anatomy, histology, physiology, biochemistry, public health, and nutrition.

Third year: Pathological anatomy, parasitology and general diseases, microbiology, pharmacology, clinical pathology, public health, nutrition, and psychiatry. Clinical introductory lectures are given in pathological physiology, internal medicine, surgery, obstetrics and gynecology, pediatrics, neurology, and psychiatry.

Fourth year: Internal medicine, surgery, obstetrics and gynecology, pediatrics, neurology, psychiatry, public health, and nutrition. Introductory lectures are given in ophthalmology, dermato-venereology; otorhinolaryngology, dentistry and oral diseases, radiology, and pharmacology.

Fifth year: Pediatrics, neurology, psychiatry, ophthalmology, dermato-venereology, otorhinolaryngology, dentistry and oral diseases, radiology, and pharmacology.

Sixth year: Internal medicine, surgery, obstetrics and gynecology, public health, including nutrition, and forensic medicine. Included in internal medicine are cardiology, pulmonary diseases, tropical diseases, endocrinology, and psychosomatic disorders.

Material given in the introductory lectures is not subject to examination.

The Students

The University of Indonesia medical school receives close to 4,000 applications a year from which it must select 200 students. Currently there are 1,202 medical students enrolled, with an average of about 200 in each class. It graduates about 150 students a year, while the other ten schools graduate a total of about 100.

Indonesian medical students have always been in the front lines: in the nationalist movement during Dutch domination, during the Japanese occupation, in the independence war following World War II and, last but not least, during the student rebellion early in 1966 when they, together with other university students and school children, supported by the army, toppled the pro-Communist Sukarno régime virtually overnight.

During the three months of the student demonstrations the historic medical school building at Salemba served as their headquarters. The first death to occur in front of the Presidential Palace was that of a fourth-year medical student, Arief Rachman Hakim, who became a national hero; millions of Indonesians attended his funeral.

Contrary to the situation in most other countries, medical students in Indonesia are not causing any trouble at the present time. This may be due to recent history when students and faculty worked together in the effort to unseat Sukarno. The students are critical about certain aspects of medical school, such as the way their teachers present lectures, but they do not interfere in matters of curriculum.

Changes in the Curriculum

In 1966 the entire Faculty of Medicine of the University of Indonesia held a meeting with the purpose of making a thorough review of the curriculum, defining more clearly the aims of the faculty. The meeting was attended by a delegation of students.

Among other matters the conference resolved to agree on the following:

1. To improve the curriculum by integrating the teaching of clinical and related subjects and to promote educational measures for the evaluation of teaching methods.

2. To introduce medical ethics and religion as part of the curricuum.

3. To promote activities that would stimulate the students' sense of dedication to their people and the country, such as participating in field work within the framework of the teaching of public health, nutrition, and family planning.

4. To define the aims and purposes of the faculty as follows: "The Faculty of Medicine, University of Indonesia, aims and strives to educate medical doctors who are dedicated to the nation's ideology of *Pantjasila,* competent and capable to practice and develop the medical sciences in the widest sense of the word, conscious of the prevailing conditions in Indonesia, and thoroughly mindful of the oath of Hippocrates."

DAIZO USHIBA
Professor and Head of Education
Department of Microbiology
Keio University
School of Medicine
Keio, Japan

JAPAN

Recent Changes in Medical Education

The system of medical education in Japan changed considerably in 1968 with the abolition of internships. While this change came about mainly due to widespread pressure from students, the internship system had had a complicated history.

Under the guidance of the United States, the internship was established in Japan immediately after World War II. Unfortunately, however, it did not develop as expected and during the twenty-odd-year period, especially in recent years, dissatisfaction and protests against the prevailing conditions increased among the students. The wave of student protests even invaded some schools where the system had been practiced rather effectively.

The students' dissatisfaction was focused on the bureaucratic administration which they accused of not giving enough support to interns in terms of teaching facilities, salaries, living conditions, and other perquisites. Although the same unhappiness was voiced by the teachers, the reason for the failure of the internship system may be attributed both to bureaucracy and to teachers. Unfortunately, there has been a tradition in Japan for faculty to put more emphasis on research than on teaching, although this situation is changing rapidly. Medical faculty members had lacked enthusiasm and had made little effort to improve education in general.

Result of the Change—the "Reported Doctor" System

The unrest of several years duration reached a climax in the spring of 1968, and as a result the Medical Practitioner's Law was revised.

Daizo Ushiba received his M.D. from Keio University School of Medicine in 1936 and the Med.Sc.D. in 1941. From 1947 to 1965 he was professor and chairman of the Department of Microbiology at Keio and was dean of the medical school from 1965 to 1969. He is presently professor and head of education in the Department of Microbiology at the university. Dr. Ushiba was unable to attend the conference.

Under the revised law medical school graduates are able to obtain a license to practice after they pass the national board examination that is held immediately following their graduation.

What, then, was substituted in the place of internship? Many arguments on this subject occur, particularly concerning the obligation to take postgraduate training. Here again, because of pressure from the students the compulsory postgraduate system was rejected and there remains only a mutilated provision under which the directors of qualified teaching hospitals report to the government the names of trainees who have finished a special two-year course.

This noncompulsory registration, or "reported doctor" system as we call it, might be considered to be meaningless. However, although it is not fully supported by the medical profession it does have some merit in that for the first time in history the government has a budget for the postgraduate training of doctors, and every teaching hospital, whether national, prefectural, municipal, or private, can obtain funds according to the number of applicants it accepts for training. This represents a major advance, considering the government's hitherto cool attitude toward medical education.

In spite of this merit, however, the law is again facing strong resistance. This time the situation is more complicated; protests are coming in not only from students but from faculty members, particularly in national medical schools, who are criticizing the government's poor budgeting. There is a presentiment that the history of the internship system may be repeated. This time, however, the students' protests are more clearly political and are directed toward the national medical care system or, in their words, the cheap labor for medical care in the teaching hospitals that is provided for under the law.

The Undergraduate Curriculum

In Japan students are qualified to enter medical school after completing twelve years of education—six years in primary school and three each in middle and high schools. Medical school entrance examinations are usually highly competitive; in 1968 only 6.8 per cent of the applicants could be admitted (see Table 1). Students may apply to several schools in the same year. In any given year about half the applicants to the more prestigious universities may be taking the entrance examinations for the second, third, or even fourth time after having failed the previous time. This keen competition for admission and the relatively low dropout rate after admission are characteristic of Japanese medical education.

TABLE 1. APPLICANTS AND ADMITTED STUDENTS IN JAPANESE MEDICAL SCHOOLS IN 1968

	Number of schools	Number of applicants	Number of admitted students	Percentage admitted
National schools	24	28,078	2,367	8.4
Prefectural and municipal schools	9	14,668	636	4.3
Private schools	13	21,446	1,367	6.4
Total	46	64,192	4,370	6.8

At present the undergraduate course is divided into two years of premedical and four years of medical studies. Subjects in the premedical period are decided upon principally by the Ministry of Education (see Table 2). In each division certain credits must be taken; the selection of subjects in the humanities and social science divisions is optional.

For the four-year medical curriculum the Ministry of Education has established so-called standard hours of medical education that specify the total teaching hours and the percentage of time to be spent on each subject (see Table 3). Although the standard is purported to be merely a recommendation, naturally, it has acted as a bureaucratic pressure and the curriculum in all medical school has generally followed along this line in the past few years. As a result, our curriculum is rather crowded, and, in addition, more hours are spent in didactic teaching than in laboratory work in accordance with the traditional German system that was introduced to Japan more than 100 years ago.

The governmental standard has sometimes acted as a hindrance to the medical schools in revising their curricula. Nevertheless, during the past few years several medical schools have made rather extensive reforms in their teaching methods. For example, innovations introduced

TABLE 2. THE PREMEDICAL CURRICULUM

1. *Subjects in General Cultural Education*

   Humanities Division: philosophy, ethics, history, literature
   Social Sciences Division: law, sociology, politics, economics
   Natural Sciences Division: physics, chemistry, biology (including experimental work)

2. *Fundamental Subjects*
   Mathematics and some advanced studies in the natural sciences
3. *Foreign Languages*
   Either English and German or English and French (another language may be substituted for one of these combinations)
4. *Health and Physical Culture* (lecture and practice)

TABLE 3. STANDARD HOURS IN THE CURRICULUM RECOMMENDED BY THE MINISTRY OF EDUCATION

Course	% of hours
Medicine	20
Surgery	10
Anatomy	9
Electives	6
Physiology	6
Pathology	6
Biochemistry	4
Microbiology	4
Obstetrics and gynecology	4
Pharmacology	4
Pediatrics	3
Public Health	3
Dermatology	2
Hygiene	2
Legal Medicine	2
Ophthalmology	2
Orthopedics	2
Otorhinolaryngology	2
Parasitology	2
Psychiatry	2
Radiology	2
Urology	2
Anesthesiology	1

Note: There are over 35 course hours a week, 30 weeks a year, totaling 4,200 hours over the 4-year period. Less than 600 hours may be added.

Electives shall be in medical psychology, medical history, hospital and medical administration, rehabilitation, basic radiological medicine, nutrition, oral surgery, etc., or clinical or research work.

into the curriculum include an emphasis on laboratory work in basic medicine that parallels that on lectures, joint lectures in basic and clinical subjects, clinico-pathological conferences, small-group bedside teaching, and clinical clerkships. Since the abolition of the internships last year, almost the entire fourth year in many schools is now being spent in bedside teaching and polyclinics. But no extensive modification of the curriculum or experimental studies on its reformation have ever been made.

POSTGRADUATE MEDICAL TRAINING

After the war, along with the introduction of internships, another new feature of medical education was the establishment of postgraduate medical schools. The postgraduate courses usually cover five major fields—physiology, pathology, social medicine, internal medicine, and surgery—each of which is further subdivided into several specialties. After graduating from medical school, a candidate for postgraduate training must pass an entrance examination and acquire a specified number of credits in one of the above-mentioned courses over a period of four years. He is then qualified to submit a dissertation in order to obtain the degree of "Igaku-Hakushi" (Doctor of Medical Science). This degree may also be obtained without attending school, through the presentation of a doctoral dissertation, but more than five years' research in a particular field is required in this case.

There is much criticism of the postgraduate school system, particularly of the poor staffing and inadequate facilities. Moreover, the distinction between the clinical course in postgraduate school and the specialty course in clinical medicine, which has just been started under specified programs, is becoming vague. Reconsideration of this system is urgently needed.

Future Outlook

It is very difficult at present to comment on the prospects of medical education in Japan. The direction of the reforms seems to have two facets: the reform of the educational system and the reform of educational methods or curriculum. Japan has to face both facets simultaneously, which will certainly take a long time.

With these problems in mind, I recently proposed the establishment of a nationwide organization that would sponsor scientific meetings to discuss medical education and publish a journal specializing in medical education. To my delight, the Japan Society of Medical Education has been inaugurated and has many supporters. It is hoped that this society will become an important element in promoting the future reform of medical education in Japan.

PREM N. WAHI
Director General
Indian Council of Medical Research
New Delhi, India

INDIA

IN RECENT YEARS medical education in India has been undergoing critical evaluation from the point of view of whether it is preparing physicians best suited to serve our developing but dynamic society and whether it is competent to keep abreast of the rapid advances in scientific knowledge. The constant desire and endeavor to revise and improve medical education has been further intensified by the increase in international contacts at both the student and faculty levels.

The physician-to-population ratio in India is 1:5,800, but this does not give a true picture of the situation as most of the physicians are concentrated in urban areas. The ratio in the villages is only about 1:30,000 population. An increase in the production of doctors has thus become imperative, and efforts to achieve this at the national level are twofold: building additional medical colleges and increasing the intake in individual institutions.

India has 94 medical colleges that admit 11,000 students annually; total enrollment is between 65,000 and 70,000. Almost 10,000 physicians are qualified each year. At present, we have 86,000 physicians and 240,000 hospital beds.

The opening of new medical colleges without a simultaneous expansion of teaching and research facilities in the existing institutions has necessitated the recruitment of staff with little experience, especially in nonclinical subjects. Existing colleges have insisted on increasing their output of physicians without expanding the physical and

---

Prem N. Wahi received his medical degree from the University of Lucknow in 1932. His postgraduate work was done at Lucknow, at the London Hospital Medical College, and at the New England Deaconess Hospital in Boston. He was professor and head of the Department of Pathology and dean of the Faculty of Medicine at the University of Lucknow until 1968 when he was appointed vice chancellor of Agra University. In 1969 he became director general of the Indian Council of Medical Research. He is a fellow of the Royal College of Physicians (London), of the National Academy of Sciences, and the Academy of Medical Sciences in India, and of the International Academy of Cytology. Dr. Wahi was unable to attend the conference.

academic facilities, and this quantitative expansion has lowered the quality of education to a certain extent. Although the faculties desire to adhere to the highest possible standards, the dilemma of quality versus quantity has reached dramatic proportions.

Admissions Procedures

To qualify for admission to medical college in India a student must be seventeen years of age and have had eleven years of elementary and high school education and one year of pre-university education.

There is a wide disparity between the various methods employed for the selection of candidates. Many institutions hold an admissions test and select students in an open competition. The subjects prescribed for the test differ slightly from place to place, but by and large they are physics, chemistry, and biology. Another procedure is to select candidates on the basis of the grades obtained at the qualifying examination. At most institutions there is no test to judge the aptitude of the candidates. It is generally felt that existing methods of selection are defective, placing too much emphasis on scholastic achievement and none on the candidate's personality as a contributing factor to his qualifications as a doctor.

Curriculum

The present medical course runs for four and one-half years followed by one year of compulsory internship. The first one and one-half years are devoted to preclinical subjects—anatomy, physiology, and biochemistry. In the following three years the students study pharmacology, pathology, microbiology, forensic medicine, preventive and social medicine, surgery, medicine, ophthalmology, and obstetrics and gynecology. After successfully completing these courses, the students work as interns for one year in a recognized hospital, spending three-month periods each in medicine, surgery, obstetrics and gynecology, and preventive and social medicine. The latter three months are spent in a rural primary health center. On completion of the internship the students are awarded the degree of M.B., B.S. (Bachelor of Medicine, Bachelor of Surgery) .

Assessment of Students

The traditional methods of examining medical students are still practiced by means of a series of professional examinations consisting of written papers and practical, clinical, and oral tests. The written papers are of the essay type, questions and answers.

The first professional examination covers anatomy, physiology, and biochemistry, and the candidate must pass it in order to qualify for clinical training. The second professional examination includes pharmacology, forensic medicine, pathology, and microbiology. The final examination covers preventive and social medicine, surgery, ophthalmology, and obstetrics and gynecology. The three professional examinations are given one and one-half years apart and are held twice a year. An average of 20 to 40 per cent of the students fail in these examinations.

In most universities no recognition is given to the day-to-day classwork of the students. The medical colleges hold sessional examinations, and in some faculties a percentage of marks obtained therein are counted toward university results.

The maintenance of minimum standards in undergraduate education is ensured by periodic inspections held by the Medical Council of India, a statutory body appointed by the Parliament. The regulation of courses, details of curriculum, and formulation of standards, are primarily the functions of the universities, through their faculties of medicine and boards of studies.

Recent Trends

In recent years some interesting developments have occurred in medical education in India. Substantial reforms have been implemented by the Medical Council of India, the Indian Association for Advancement of Medical Education, the Indian Academy of Medical Sciences, and the Indian Council of Medical Research, through its expert committees on research in medical education and health practices. These bodies have also helped to increase communication between the Indian medical colleges.

Premedical Education

Premedical education is facing a serious problem due to the recent reorganization of secondary education. The provision of a higher secondary course in place of the old intermediate science course does not provide prospective medical students with an appropriate educational background. Some faculties have already introduced a premedical course, extending over a period of one year prior to admission to the medical course, thus making it a part of the first-year medical curriculum and extending the medical training by one year. The question of curriculum content in such a course and the role of universities in such a training program are other important aspects under consideration. The tendency is to make these courses broad-based by including such subjects as humanities, medical statistics, and human genetics, in addition to physics, chemistry, mathematics, and biology.

Medical Curriculum

Indian medical educators accept the fact that changes in the traditional medical curriculum are desirable and, indeed, necessary. Medical education is dynamic, and the rapidly expanding core of new information is producing a crowded curriculum. Unfortunately, all attempts at reforms have been piecemeal and half-hearted and have succeeded only in adding to the already over-burdened curriculum.

Medical education needs a complete "new look" in order for it to fulfill its goal of enabling the student to acquire medical knowledge, to develop attitudes that will enable him to see his patients as whole individuals, to serve the community as well as the individual patient, and to effectively serve a society that is predominantly rural and changing rapidly. Most medical faculties now have committees that are constantly reviewing existing curricula and gearing them to the changing needs of medical education.

To achieve this objective both curriculum content and educational methods are under constant scrutiny. The purpose of any reorientation of educational programs should be to produce a physician who is able to fulfill his mission in a society where total health has now become a national concern rather than the concern of the individual.

The population pyramid of a developing country such as India has a broad base; there are a large number of young people and a relatively small number of old people, with the result that geriatric needs are not yet predominant. Furthermore, a high percentage of the population live in the rural areas. With increasing industrialization, social changes are taking place rather rapidly, which make it all the more obligatory for medical education to prepare physicians to adapt themselves to changing circumstances and disease patterns. Accelerated urbanization is producing, and will continue to produce, very serious physical, mental, and social health problems in developing countries.

Although pediatrics is at present more important in India than geriatrics, with the control of communicable diseases, the reduction of infant mortality, and the availability of better diagnosis and treatment, life expectancy is going to rise. The current trend is toward an increase in degenerative diseases, such as cardiovascular disorders. Also to be reckoned with are the hazards associated with rapid industrialization and the consequent urbanization of the population.

These are some of the developments that are already effecting changes in health care needs in India.

Medical education should aim to produce a physician who can tackle these individual problems successfully, while at the same time preparing him for the unknown needs of the future that will result from the fast-changing social complex and the expanding pool of medical knowledge. Unfortunately, medical educators are not taking cognizance of the trends with which the students will have to cope later on. The concept of continuing education is, however, fundamental for the future of medical care in the developing countries.

Pediatric care is receiving due recognition, and separate departments equipped for training and research are now to be found in almost all medical colleges. Preventive pediatrics and child nutrition are important components in the training and service programs. Pediatric research is making a significant contribution and is primarily responsible for the steady decline in infant mortality.

A good deal of attention has been given to preventive and social medicine in recent years, and the teaching of this dicipline has been integrated throughout the medical curriculum. Compared to its status in western countries, however, much has yet to be achieved. There is a noticeable tendency to move away from the old, established, clinically oriented training pattern toward field training in block hospitals and rural health centers. Three months of the internship year is devoted to such programs, thus further enhancing the value of the training.

The community in which the field work is carried out is usually part of a larger community from which the teaching hospital draws its patients. The purpose of such programs is to introduce the student to the practice of comprehensive medicine in his clinical years and to expose him to the kind of rural society in which he may be required to serve after graduation.

Among the disciplines that are gradually being introduced into the curriculum are medical statistics, humanities, psychiatry, psychological medicine, and human genetics. Too little attention is being given to medical statistics at the undergraduate level, and there is a growing realization that it should be taught early in the medical course. Genetics is another discipline that has been completely ignored until recently, and in some institutions it is now being taught as an integrated course. The anatomy course includes basic genetics and, later on, each department teaches the subject as it relates to its own field. Similarly, the teaching of psychiatry is gaining momentum and the tendency is to clearly integrate it with preventive and social medicine in order to enable the students to observe people's behavior in their normal environment.

Educational Methodology

In recent years considerable concern has been voiced over the techniques of medical education. At present it is primarily academic, even though time is allotted for practical work. But even the practical training is more theoretical than otherwise. The existing pattern of medical education fails to provide the student with an opportunity to discover himself, with the result that he is given unrealistic motivational concepts. The student's learning process is to a considerable degree affected by his motivation. Medical faculties in India are, therefore, reorganizing their educational programs in order to consider not only how to produce a competent physician but how to produce one who will continue to contribute to the art of medicine, who will be actively interested in the progress of medical research, and who will be able to handle successfully the ever-arising problems in medicine. He should be equipped intellectually to approach all future problems as a scientist and research scholar imbued with the spirit of critical evaluation. To do so he must have considerable independence, the habit of logical thinking, a sense of responsibility and initiative, and a sound knowledge of the subject involved.

The present medical curriculum, based on the old authoritarian approach of set lectures and demonstrations accompanied by didactic teaching, is being replaced by techniques that encourage self-education, such as small-group projects, conferences, seminars, and tutorials in which the students are major participants. Another meaningful change is the provision of elective time that allows the student to browse around on his own. During this time he is encouraged to work on research projects in basic science departments. Another successful training procedure is the introduction of experimental methods whereby a student learns the process of a disease by studying at least one subject in depth and performing experiments. This helps to educate him in scientific methods of thinking and inculcate in him curiosity and initiative.

Exposing the undergraduates to research methodology and encouraging those who show an aptitude for it to work on departmental research programs will help them to develop a critical faculty that will enable them to appraise the effectiveness of medical services. While the emphasis on operational research has a low priority compared to training in diagnostic, curative, and preventive aspects of disease, such an exposure, however minimum it might be, will motivate the student to keep abreast of advances in medicine and help him to evaluate the newer data.

Some faculties have introduced integrated or correlated teaching programs into the curriculum, and this is a step in the right direction, as it will not only help to shorten the syllabus but make it possible to produce a physician capable of viewing the patient as a whole. Due to a shortage of teachers, however, this has not been successfully implemented in any institution that I know of. It has not yet been decided whether the end results warrant the additional expenditure required for staff salaries. Interdepartmental co-operation is still favored over closely integrated teaching. In the newer colleges, multidiscipline laboratories are being established.

Examination Reforms

All medical educators recognize the necessity for reforms in the examination system, and experiments are being carried out on newer methods which some faculties have adopted. The conventional methods, with their greater subjective element and inherent limitations, are still accepted procedure in most institutions. Some faculties prefer objective examination techniques to the traditional, time-consuming, question-and-answer, essay-type examination, but in the face of the teacher shortage the amount of time required to design questions has been a deterrent to adopting this system. Day-to-day assessment and frequent sessional examinations are being used more and more, and multiple-choice tests are being introduced which are considered economical in terms of faculty time; at present both types of examination techniques are being employed.

The changing pattern of medical education in India still falls far short of producing the ideal physician, who will serve the needs of society and contribute leadership to the community. Still it is going in the right direction to produce a physician who can more effectively fulfill his role under changing circumstances.

An additional handicap to progress is the lack of competent medical administrators to organize and create a proper educational atmosphere. Medical education administration has not received due recognition in India, with the result that the productivity of our institutions, in terms of both quality of manpower and scientific contributions, leaves much to be desired.

With its limited resources, the primary objective of a developing country such as India—to provide the benefits of modern medicine to its predominantly rural population—has yet to be achieved. The key factors to be reckoned with, in terms of the physician working in the rural areas, are the absence of physical and professional facilities, unsatisfactory living conditions, cultural isolation, the reluctance to exchange urban amenities for physical discomforts, and the absence of compensatory incentives. Unless solutions are found to these problems all the benefits of improvements in medical education will still be available only to the 20 per cent of the population living in the cities of India.

LOWELL T. COGGESHALL

The Coggeshall Report: A Summary

The enormous expansion of medical education, research, and patient care over the past twenty years has created serious problems in every country. Of the many acute problems the most basic and, in the long run, the most important are those facing medical educators. How can existing institutions produce a sufficient number of qualified physicians capable of operating an effective, comprehensive, medical-care delivery system at a price society can afford?

The deans of medical faculties in the United States, with the support of the Association of American Medical Colleges (A.A.M.C.) decided to examine in some detail the following question: Are current methods and practices, designed to provide health personnel of all categories, and existing or planned programs and facilities adequate to meet our present and future national needs? A committee I had the honor to chair attempted to find an answer. The membership was composed of President Clark Kerr of the University of California, Dean William Hubbard of the University of Michigan Medical School; Professor Michael De Bakey of Baylor Medical College; Dean John Deitrich of Cornell University Medical College; and Professor George Perera of Columbia University College of Physicians and Surgeons. We were to investigate the future development of medical education and determine the role that the A.A.M.C. should play, if necessary, in the decades ahead.

It was agreed at the outset that no valid and convincing judgments could be reached without first reviewing the broader aspects of medical

---

Lowell T. Coggeshall was born in Indiana and received his M.D. from Indiana University School of Medicine in 1928. He became assistant professor of medicine at the University of Chicago in that same year. He served as a captain in the United States Navy during World War II. In 1946 he was appointed chairman of the Department of Medicine at Chicago, in 1957 dean of the Division of Biological Sciences, and in 1961 vice president of the university, a post from which he has since retired. The "Coggeshall report" was published in 1965 by the Association of American Medical Colleges.

education, research, and service. The report of this survey, published in 1965, entitled "Planning for Medical Progress Through Education" (usually referred to as the Coggeshall Report) is relevant wherever there is concern about the future development of medical education. I shall mention only a few aspects of that survey that seem to be pertinent to the topic of this conference.

The study was based primarily upon the authoritative opinions of a great many people who exert influence over or are concerned about medical education. Specifically they included members of Congress, government executives, governors, executives of Blue Cross, insurance companies, pharmaceutical companies, foundations, representatives of specialty boards and other professional organizations, and leading educators, university presidents, deans, medical faculties, and students.

From the beginning the survey elicited a surprising unanimity of concern; few persons interviewed believed that the improvements needed were matters of minor adjustment. The general opinion was that there were many serious problems in need of immediate attention. Some held that our system of medical education needed radical adjustment because it was geared to the past rather than to the future.

I shall sketch briefly the background that confronted the committee. Until the early 1900's, physicians in the United States were trained largely by reading and apprenticeship, and medicine was beginning to be held in low esteem because of the activities of so many poorly trained doctors. Suddenly many new schools appeared, small and large, established by those who wished to raise the standards of medical education. In addition, many proprietary schools were organized for profit.

The Flexner Report issued in 1910 revealed a shocking disparity in the quality of the then more than 135 schools—no admission requirements other than an inferior formal education and payment of an entrance fee; little or no instruction from poorly trained teachers, and so forth. The report focused its concern on three areas: (1) stringent concern over all standards for admission and instruction; (2) the importance of relating medical education to the universities' curricula; and (3) the need to provide full-time faculty in laboratories and hospitals.

Subsequently, new laws were enacted in many states and more than half of the existing schools were forced to close because they were unable to meet the new standards. The seventy-five remaining schools settled down to a fairly routine existence, making few changes until the outbreak of World War II. Until that time most curricula were overloaded with lectures emphasizing diagnosis and treatment. Students were not permitted to have contact with patients until the last year or two of medical school. After graduation most went directly into practice without having had an internship.

As the specialty boards came into existence this custom changed gradually so that by 1940 most students were taking internships and serving an additional three to five years in specialized training in order to satisfy the requirements of their particular discipline. Medical research was conducted almost entirely in the very few schools that had private endowments.

The educational process gradually improved, largely through the efforts of the A.A.M.C. and the American Medical Association, which established educational standards for member schools and maintained periodic accreditation reviews of their performance.

The events that followed the war demonstrated conclusively that the previous pattern of medical education would not be able to adjust to the variety of new external forces that were appearing rapidly.

The most substantive changes that occurred in those years were of qualitative importance. Medical education increased greatly in complexity and it became necessary to teach more than diagnosis and treatment. Mere expertise in personal diagnostic and prognostic skills was no longer sufficient. Chemotherapeutic advances and many new discoveries gradually placed the well-trained physician on the offensive. It was no longer possible for the physician to practice on an independent physician-patient basis. He had to cope with the many new internal and external forces and trends that for the most part had materialized since 1945.

Our committee sought to identify the most significant trends that were influencing the patterns of medical education and altering the practice of medicine. I shall attempt to identify them briefly.

Scientific Advances. The discovery of antibiotics to control infection is a striking example, and their usage literally changed medical practice overnight. Subsequent great advances included the latest spectacular and highly publicized organ transplants. The aggregate result of these advances drastically altered the educational needs of the student and placed special emphasis on improving the quality of postgraduate medical education as the physician became a much more positive factor in preventive and curative medicine.

Population Changes. Although outside the area of health care, the explosive growth, changing composition, and distribution of the population has a profound implication for health educators. In the United

States our population has grown from 76 million in 1900 to an estimated 200 million or more by 1970. More significant is the constantly increasing percentage of persons in the upper age groups where disease is more prevalent, more chronic in nature, more refractory to treatment, and associated with more social problems. The worldwide population has become much more mobile and the task of preparing physicians to care for the hordes crowding into the urban areas is becoming increasingly difficult.

Increasing Health Expectation. Throughout history man has been conditioned to accept illness, plagues, and personal injury as normal. Today, however, medical advances are announced with great frequency and people are becoming accustomed to expect good health care and will travel any distance to get it. There is an increasing awareness of the value of preventive medicine—it is no longer necessary to force a community into an immunization program. Changing expectations have certainly produced a continuing and profound effect on the way health care is delivered as well as on the kind and amount that people seek.

Increasingly Effective Demand for Health Care. Basically, people are now familiar with the competency or the training of their physicians and appreciate the value of the health care that is available. Through private or public resources they are for the first time able to pay for such care, and hence they are making more effective demands. Over 80 per cent of the civilian population in the United States is covered by some form of health prepayment and legislation for broader coverage is inevitable. The demand is growing louder as more and more people find it increasingly difficult to find a doctor.

Increasing Specialization. Over 85 per cent of the graduating physicians plan to become specialists. While the rise of specialization has improved the quality of medical care for those to whom it is available, qualitatively and quantitatively it is creating problems for the medical schools. As each specialty gradually increases its educational requirements the training falls primarily on the shoulders of medical school faculties in the teaching hospitals, usually without initial discussion or planning by the deans and their advisors. Even subspecialization is now occurring among the supportive skills of medicine.

Although specialization is creating a higher grade of medical care, it is driving out the general practitioner. It is contributing greatly to the institutionalization of medical practice, to the need for a "team care" approach with more health personnel of all types. Team care, largely through clinics, is a rapidly growing trend as the individual practitioner gradually disappears from the scene, and this is causing medical school faculties to reorient their planning and practices to meet the needs of a more demanding public.

Increasing Development of Technological Advances and Equipment. Surgery, radiology, and diagnostic laboratories, especially, are utilizing a veritable spawn of new devices that are profoundly altering the practice of medicine, the education of the physician, and, particularly, the training of nurses and technicians. Of great significance will be the rapid adaptation of the computer to all aspects of medical education and practice.

Increasing Institutionalization of Health Care. This is arising from the chronic shortage of physicians, the trend toward specialization, new advances in science, population concentrations, and rising health expectations. The average physician has neither the skills nor the equipment in his office for other than the most routine care. In urban areas, especially, emergency clinics are being inundated by patients who have learned that this is the only place where medical care is available.

The Growing Need for Manpower. If one includes the college years, the training of a physician now takes from nine to fifteen years or even longer. It takes six to seven years to train his supporting staff. Much of the time required for the physician's training is now spent in extensive research programs; some believe that too much emphasis is placed on research during the student years. In the United States it is becoming quite evident that we are far from producing an adequate supply of medical talent, despite considerable pressure to do so. Progress has been made in that new medical schools are being established and admissions are being increased in all schools, but we must admit to a probably constant inability to produce a sufficient number of physicians. The alternative is to place greater reliance on a system that will generate more health associates and assistants.

The Cost of Medical Care. The rising cost of health care is compounding the problems of the medical educational system. Health service will soon be our nation's largest industry. In 1968 more than $53 billion was spent on services and nearly $2 billion for research. Average daily hospital bed costs are nearing $100. And yet it is generally accepted that a large number of our citizens receive almost no medical care.

These costs are threatening the very existence of the private medical schools as they attempt to provide faculty and facilities for their enormous responsibilities.

The Expanding Role of Government. The last major trend is the government's increasing participation in medical education, research, and service—this is an irreversible phenomenon.

The committee believed that the implications of the foregoing trends made it clear that medical education was in need of reforms and that the A.A.M.C., particularly, could play a leading role in initiating them. It was evident that the medical schools needed to pay more attention to the requirements of the nation and of the community for health care and personnel, not only for the brief span of four years, as was the custom for most schools. Many more and better trained physicians and supportive personnel had to be provided.

The national development of an improved if not entirely new health system is a pressing need. Walter McNerney, President of the Blue Cross Association of America, has stated that the evocative question of whether the United States needs a new health system should be taken seriously. Medical education in the future should be planned as a continuum—a continuing process under co-ordinated leadership. There must be a greater emphasis on interdisciplinary relationships, particularly between research and instruction. Most important, the university should assume greater responsibility for education for health and medical sciences.

The purpose of the report's many recommendations was to prepare the A.A.M.C. to play a greater leadership role in the future. It was believed imperative for one organization to either direct or co-ordinate the many fragmented efforts now controlling the destiny of American medical education.

The committee believed that the findings clearly demonstrated that the present system of medical education was outmoded and should be reoriented in order to meet society's need for medical talent to provide adequate medical care. It also held that the evidence was indubitably in favor of the university's breaking its traditional concept of regarding the medical school as a unit solely concerned with four years of undergraduate education.

Finally, it was convinced that medical school faculties in turn should play a leadership role in helping solve the health needs of the community and the nation, rather than limiting their concern to curative medicine within the comfortable four walls of their teaching hospitals.

The survey offered many broad and specific recommendations on philosophy, objectives, programs, services, organizations, relationships, facilities, and financing. In my opinion the most significant of these was that the university accept the responsibility for providing medical education as a continuum, for only then can education and research be successfully integrated. Second, that the A.A.M.C., the only organization capable of guiding medical education through the difficult years ahead, should reorganize itself so as to accept the challenge.

What has been the impact of the report? The chairman of the committee may not be the best person to give an objective evaluation, but one observation indicative of the interest it aroused is that in excess of 25,000 copies have been requested from all over the world.

The A.A.M.C. accepted most of the suggested plans for its reorganization. Rather than remain an organization composed solely of medical deans it is now subdivided into three councils—A Council of Deans, a Council of Academic Societies, and a Council of Teaching Hospitals. This alone has given the A.A.M.C. great vigor, and a sense of purpose and progress is now evident.

At the risk of appearing immodest, may I conclude by quoting Dr. William Anlyan, the first chairman of the Council of Deans, who reported on the impact of the Coggeshall Report at the annual meeting of our Council on Medical Education this year: "It can be stated that in less than four years the A.A.M.C. has undergone a major evolutionary change triggered by the Coggeshall Report of April 1965. The organization is now truly representative of the major components of academic medical centers. It has visible and vibrant interfaces with the affairs of other educational and research components in the nation, the Federal Government, the American Medical Association, and the practicing physician, the medical student, the college student, and perhaps most important of all the society and the American people whom we serve."

We are a long way from solving the many problems facing us in medical education today, but I am proud of the committee's efforts which I am convinced outlined a definitive course for future action and improvement.

Panel: The Medical Students

Introduction

DR. GALLEGO: Present-day university students may be regarded from two complementary points of view:

1) As members of a generation caught up in the general movement of modern youth; and

2) As individuals concerned with the problems, specific anxieties, and aspirations common to all students.

The students' social attitude is one of rebellion and universal examination of conscience, resulting in a strengthening of their class consciousness. The universal revolt of the young reflects an intellectual malaise that is not new to them. What is new is the violent revolutionary manner in which it is being expressed.

Students are rebelling against an immediate reality that affects their daily lives, namely, the structure, organization, content, and method of university teaching. They show toward their own professional prospects—and the possibilities of social integration—a growing anxiety about the organization of a society that must absorb them, but whose ideology they reject. This creates in them a state of uncertainty as to the objectives of that society beyond purely material satisfactions.

Young intellectuals have always approached the society in which they are to participate with reforming zeal. In the past they were impelled by a national consciousness; the problems they had to live with were limited in range, being either local or national in character. They saw the solutions in various revolutionary ideologies that for the most part were in a phase of theoretical development or early practical application.

Two factors have changed these reactions, broadening them and giving them a new focus. On the one hand, modern communications techniques have brought to the level of universal consciousness what previous generations saw as merely local problems. On the other hand, modern youth is the most sensitive witness to the failure of the ideologies that dominated the thinking of their predecessors who saw in them the solutions for their social experience.

In this climate of universality the young rebels today reject alike the Vietnam war and the invasion of Czechoslovakia. Contrary to what the "respectable" men in both the East and West believe, the young Americans who avoid military service are not "communists" or "foreign agents," any more than the young Czechs who oppose their government and the Soviet invasion of their country are "agents of Yankee imperialism."

The students' ideological position, both anti-capitalist and anti-Marxist–Leninist, is what gives international cohesion to the rebel youth movement. They seek socialization and individual freedom. They are at one and the same time Marxists and trans-Marxists. This leads them to reject the "consumption society," to refuse to be formed in only one dimension, and to oppose Marxism–Leninism. This phenomenon among the youth of the world is most interesting.

For the young rebels, Soviet communism has become the collaborator of Western neocapitalism, renouncing the revolution and becoming imperialist itself, and using the same methods in its international commercial relations. It identifies itself with neocapitalism when it collaborates in the maintenance of the authoritarian state ruled by an "elite" or "apparat" and uses the same kind of physical and intellectual repression of the masses.

The revolt of the young began years ago in several countries, even before they were aware of the existence of the theorists of the anti-authoritarian Left led by Herbert Marcuse. The skeptical generation of the early postwar period has been followed by a romantic generation, *Sturm und Drang*—that seeks direct action. Its popular ideological image was given by Rudi Dutschke and Daniel Cohn-Benedict whose theory is a dialectical attack on the Leninist concept of revolution based on the domination of an "elite," and whose practice relies on the spontaneity of the masses and therefore on the emergence of forms of action in the midst of a struggle whose validity is constantly re-examined.

The basic feature of Dutschke's theory is his demand for an authentic revolution from all nonhuman domination: "A policy carried out by people who have not themselves undergone an internal transformation is a manipulation by 'elites.' " He bases his revolutionary attitude on human considerations: "What unites us today is not an abstract theory of history but an existential nausea that talks of freedom and at the same time represses the needs and direct interests of individuals and of peoples fighting for their socioeconomic independence."

For the theorists of the movement, revolution is a process of self-education and self-orientation. It needs a new type of man. In an advanced capitalist society the intellectuals are the only social group capable of keeping their heads clear in a climate of growing alienation. Dutschke does not believe that the students alone can create the revolution, but he does think they can unmask the process of capitalist manipulation and that it is their duty to shake the working classes out of their lethargy and insensibility by public demonstrations and constant provocation of the establishment.

The students are given a sense of belonging to a homogeneous group by the universality of today's problems and by the new revolutionary theory that bases the revolution not on the concept of "wage-earners" but on the mental capacity of each individual at his own cultural level.

The ideological position of these young people is purely destructive; they believe that constructive solutions will emerge in the midst of the revolutionary movement, spontaneously, out of students' and workers' councils. Perhaps they confuse the anticipated improvisation for constructive action with the incompetence of the chosen planning group—the students themselves (who are, after all, an "elite")! The fact is that whereas the classical ideologies, or the fact that one belonged to a definite class, could "mark" a man for life, the essentially transitory nature of the student status in the life of an individual may condition his political, social, and ideological action only in the phase of rejection, criticism, and destruction.

When the student leaves the university, society will absorb him (or poison him, as he sees it). Thus, just as Marxism–Leninism voluntarily renounced the world revolution when confronted with evolving capitalism, so the student renounces his revolution when confronted by a society with which he "collaborates;" a society, moreover, that always is in the full process of evolution.

Hence the great value of the youth movements as accelerators, pressing for an examination of conscience, denouncing a society that, if left exclusively in the hands of the "respectable" elements who hold power, would allow them to perpetuate their exclusive status in their own interest.

Although the general picture is the same, the student movement in each country has distinct and peculiar features, depending on political and socioeconomic circumstances, among which society's reaction to the student revolution plays an important part. Confronted with acts of youthful rebellion, established authority, depending on its strength and the intelligence of those who comprise it, reacts with a wide range of policies—from dialogues with the students to violent repression.

In the face of a society they reject, the students express themselves by inhibition, participation, and violent protest. It should be admitted, however, that the great mass of students of the "turbulent generation," although in revolt against society and the representatives of authority, are prepared to participate to a greater or lesser degree in discussions of the problems affecting them and aspire to take part in the management of university centers.

I would say that only two minority groups accept a complete break with authority—the "hippies" from inhibition, and those whose definite purpose is revolutionary action. The picturesque "hippies" are an anecdotal manifestion of the self-assertiveness of rebellious youth. The groups favoring revolution seek to enlist all youth and to extend their action to other groups, particularly the working class. Whether or not revolutionary action acquires a hold on the masses of students depends in large part on the actions of these minorities and, above all, on the type of repression used against them.

That is why society's forms of reaction to the revolt of the young are of such great importance. These forms are dialogue, participation, or repression. There are two kinds of repression—internal and external. Internal repression is carried out through systematic propaganda using all the means at the disposal of established power—press, radio, television, and so on. Such repression acts on the students like systematic brain-washing which in the course of time influences the great number of students not involved in direct revolutionary action. As a prophylactic, this brain-washing tends to isolate youth in its violent aspirations.

External repression is manifested by all types of physical action including police violence with all its consequences. In many countries not a few students end up in jail. Such violent external repression usually causes the whole student group to join the revolt, at least spasmodically and temporarily.

Generally speaking, when there is no violent repression the mass of students does not participate in revolutionary action except perhaps for short periods of time. The events of May 1968 at the Sorbonne are a clear example. If instead of a containment operation, which apparently appeared weak to some people, there had been the kind of repression carried out in Mexico in the weeks before the Olympic Games, it is probable that a real revolutionary situation of unsuspected consequences would have arisen in France. The containment operation, while costly for the country, elicited a reaction not only from society but from the great majority of the students, who abandoned revolutionary action so that it became little more than a revolt.

Specific Attitudes of Medical Students

Medical students feel concerned about the organization of health services in the society that will absorb them and in which they will have to play their part. They wonder if the structure, organization, content, and methods of medical school teaching are appropriate to what they believe to be their needs.

There is a marked difference in the attitudes of students in the preclinical years and those of senior students nearing their clinical apprenticeships. In the preclinical years they are more involved in the revolt of the present generation. Their lack of appreciation of the instruction they are receiving and their anxiety about their future roles in society are accompanied by a tendency to reject that society with some vehemence.

In other faculties—political science, economics, philosophy, and the humanities in general—this tendency usually lasts throughout a student's university career. But among medical students, in the clinical years it is replaced by an intense professionalization. The medical student nearing graduation usually gives up revolutionary action and seeks instead to prepare himself to practice his profession in the most remunerative way possible.

In past generations the medical student thought almost exclusively of practicing in his own country. Only a minority whose objective was medical research had a more international outlook. Today the practice of medicine is one of the most internationalized professions and the doctor with good training can expect to practice not only in his own country but in others either more or less developed than his own.

This fact gives the medical student a universal consciousness so characteristic of the young generation and leads him to think internationally during his training with regard to the methods of instruction and the way medicine is practiced in other countries. In Spain this has created an increasing interest in learning other languages.

Students know that when graduated they will face a constantly changing medical profession whose characteristics may be influenced by:

1) Factors connected with population growth; the increase in individual health expectations and in the demand of the population for better health care;

2) Increasing specialization in medical practice; the team approach to health care; and the use of technologically advanced equipment;

3) Such economic factors as the progressively rising cost of medical treatment.

As a result of these factors, we have:

a) Increasingly active intervention in improving health care by governments, foundations, and other private agencies;

b) A growing movement toward the institutionalization of health care;

c) The need to increase the number of physicians and to improve the standard of their training; the need for more and better-trained paramedical personnel.

Medical students seek, in fact demand, better professional training oriented toward eventual practice. From the first years in medical school they want direct contact with patients and practical instruction. They have lost interest in or have decisively rejected theoretical teaching that they consider not directly related to the practice of medicine.

This attitude brings them into conflict with those medical schools whose structures have remained antiquated and sometimes leads to situations where violence is possible. As a result the students are asking for the following:

1) To be consulted about the organization of teaching and about changes in the curriculum;
2) The right to criticize the functions of the teaching staff;
3) Stronger emphasis on the social aspects of medical practice;
4) Apprenticeship in language courses;
5) A system of student exchanges during holiday periods;
6) Participation in the organization of patient medical care.

At the University of Madrid medical school, for example, our students are asking for:

1) Participation of interns in the operation of university hospitals;
2) Co-operation with the College of Physicians in the planning of the students' medical practice after graduation;
3) A reorganization and improvement of medical practice.

Students are unanimous about the necessity for socialized medicine, but they ask that insured patients be free to choose their own doctor and pay for his fees. In general all their aspirations are leading toward the creation of more and better-paid physicians. As a logical consequence of looking upon medical practice as a social function of major importance they are now asking, even violently, for the abolition of military service for medical students, to be replaced by some form of social service in the medical field.

A large number of students, especially those in the last years of medical school, wish to practice their profession internationally, usually with the purpose of improving the conditions of medical practice. Hence they consider emigration to countries where better conditions prevail and there is more money to be made. Many students do not intend to return home. Others consider practicing in less developed countries than their own.

The consequences of the students' attitudes are of great interest both from the professional and social points of view. In Spain, for example, their outspokenness acted as the stimulus that brought about a fundamental reform in medical teaching. Their public pressure galvanized the government into realizing the deficiencies in medical school teaching and impelled it to take steps to improve instruction and to reorganize the hospitals. These reforms were also the result of pressure from the Social Security Administration, which needs more highly-trained doctors to staff its services, particularly its specialized hospitals.

The emigration of qualified doctors is another constructive aspect of the students' aspirations. Since many countries have an evident scarcity of medical personnel, the arrival of doctors who have had a good basic training can help to solve some of these countries' health problems. The demands of students for such basic training should encourage the medical schools to adopt a curriculum with minimum standards of practical instruction that would qualify them to issue internationally valid degrees.

In summary, the medical students are participating only to a small extent in the revolt of the turbulent generation. In the last year of studies their attitude is highly professional and they have international ambitions. If these tendencies can be channeled they should be very constructive for medicine in general.

Spain

DR. GALLEGO: At the end of our Civil War the medical schools were ruled by a dean with the assistance of an advisory body of full professors called the "Claustro de Profesores." However as deans and rectors were appointed by the Ministry of Education for political reasons (and very strong ones) there were few matters left for the Claustro to consider.

At that time also it was compulsory for all students to belong to the one and only union called "Sindicato Espanol Universitario" or S.E.U., which initially was a branch of the Falangist party. Student participation in the governance of the medical schools was limited to their having three members of the S.E.U. sitting in the Claustro with the power to vote in matters of student interest (which were decided upon by the dean). The fifty or more assistant professors in a medical school had only two votes in the Claustro.

This system existed until 1955 when the student revolt started in Spain. The revolt began when a number of S.E.U. students were "sent" to make a "spontaneous" protest in front of the British Embassy and were badly beaten up by the police.

That was the start of a rebellion that is still going on today. The small per cent of student activists organized several underground groups whose membership also included Communists (both Marxist–Leninist and Maoist), Socialists, and extreme rightists. The students had two targets: to abolish the S.E.U. and to gain the right to organize themselves in their own independent and democratic way.

Demonstrations, strikes, and fights with the police made the student unrest a matter of public concern. The government decided to do away with the S.E.U. and passed a law authorizing the students to join associations that were to be organized in accordance with regulations stated in the law. These new associations were forbidden to engage in political activities, but this restriction was not recognized by the students whose ultimate goal was a political one: to participate actively in public and university life on the basis of freedom and democracy.

Since that time students have attended faculty meetings only sporadically; in most schools they have refused to attend at all.

The students' revolt became increasingly active and resulted in some schools being closed for weeks and even months. In 1968 a serious confrontation with the police created a crisis and caused the government to appoint a new Minister of Education who has drafted a new law that will bring about a great many changes in the universities.

While everybody admits that the students have made some valid criticisms their violent revolt brought about a reaction against giving them too much power. As long as the present political situation exists in Spain I cannot foresee a large student representation in the governing bodies of our universities.

The conflict between the students and the government is serious and we expect considerable trouble. I am convinced that in the coming months the students will insist on being given the same advantages that the French students demanded and got in 1968.

UNITED STATES

DR. GLASER: Let me make some general comments about medical students in the United States. Obviously it is not possible to describe in any simple way the character of 30,000 young people, but one can make some pertinent generalizations.

Our students are usually between twenty and twenty-two years of age when they come to medical school. Most of them have spent four years in college and have completed the requirements for an A.B. degree.

As a group they are from the more affluent segment of our society; a very substantial proportion comes from families with incomes above $15,000. Several factors are operative in influencing this selection. The children of the economically advantaged are more likely to attend college, an obvious prerequisite to medical school. Further, of those who finish college the students with more favorable financial backgrounds are less likely to be deterred by the additional expense of a medical education.

Particularly striking has been the small number of medical students from the so-called minority groups. Until the past year or so a very small number of medical students came from the black community and an even smaller number from the Mexican-American (or Spanish-American) community, which in some parts of the country, particularly the West and Southwest, represents a substantial percentage of the population. Almost no students have been drawn from the relatively small American Indian group.

Many schools are now engaged in vigorous recruitment of minority students—at Stanford we have increased our total enrollment by about 20 per cent, and all the increase is represented by minority students, chiefly blacks and Mexican-Americans. We view this as a forward step, albeit one that has been too slow in coming. Some of the minority students will face academic difficulties, of course, because of the defects that exist in many segments of our educational system. Many of them have attended relatively poor primary and secondary schools, some having gone to colleges where their preparation, especially in the sciences, may have been inadequate. It is worth noting that our white students have been a potent force in supporting increased minority enrollment; many of them have been outspoken in criticizing what they consider the lack of adequate progress.

To a large extent, the problems that our schools face in increasing minority enrollment are financial. It requires a significant additional budget to provide the support that minority group students need, not to mention the cost of increasing faculty-size to handle larger teaching loads. In fact, I view the latter as far less significant than the former. Students, however, perhaps partly through our failure to inform them, have no concept of what it costs to operate a medical school. They see that we have a budget measured in millions of dollars and they ask, "With all that money, do you mean to tell us you cannot take more students?"

One can make some generalizations about the student population in American medical schools today. First of all, as a group, they are very bright. They are selected from a much larger number of qualified applicants than can be accommodated at present. There are more than two applicants for each available place, and since the number of qualified applicants continues to rise the selection process becomes even more difficult.

Let me cite some figures for Stanford: in the past year (1968–69) we received approximately 1,800 applications, but could take only 64 students, plus 10 in our minority group program. I would estimate that 1,000 of the candidates merited serious consideration, and of that number almost half were clearly qualified; that is, they could have completed the requirements for the degree had they been admitted. It is not too unlikely that we could have made a random selection from the group of 400 to 500, saved much time and effort, and perhaps have come out just as well.

Since students make multiple applications, I am not suggesting that Stanford was the first choice for all 1,800; of course, it was not. Multiple applications are submitted by all students, so all schools receive far more applications than they have places. There is no question that many qualified students are not getting into medical school today. This is a major problem, all the more so because we need more physicians and should not be turning down able people who want to serve society through medicine.

Students coming into medical school today are relatively better prepared than they were fifteen years ago, and certainly better than they were in my time. This reflects an increase in the quality of education, especially in science, not only in the colleges but in the high schools, junior high schools, and even grade schools.

If one looks at the textbooks the students in our public high schools are using today, one cannot help but be impressed with the sophistication of their content. It is not surprising, therefore, that by the time they finish college our students have had a preparation that in many instances precludes the necessity of their taking certain courses, particularly in the basic sciences.

I want to emphasize that point by citing a statistic for Stanford that would apply to many other schools. We have an outstanding Department of Biochemistry whose faculty is admirably interested in teaching. Over the past two years, however, the faculty has come to the conclusion that 40 per cent of the students who enter the medical school do not need to take the standard biochemistry course. Until our curriculum changed last year, all students had to take the course even if it meant repetition, and this produced, understandably, a distinct measure of dissatisfaction.

A relatively new phenomenon in our schools has been the critical attitude of a number of medical students toward the emphasis on science in our schools. We hear from them all the time that much of basic science is "irrelevant." Despite their relatively sophisticated background in modern science, they are upset because so much emphasis is placed on biochemistry, molecular biology, and pathologic physiology. Most of us in medical education are convinced of the importance of the science base for medicine, but a fair segment of today's students consider it not only "irrelevant" but "dehumanizing" (the latter is another word we hear a great deal).

They express the view that in American medical schools we are only interested in people with exotic or life-threatening diseases. I have to agree with them when they point out, for example, that they see many more patients with lupus erythematosus or, in the case of our university hospital, patients admitted for open-heart surgery than patients with the more common ailments that the majority of physicians see in their practice. They consider the university hospital of limited value as the locus for preparing for a medical career.

The byproduct of this situation is that some of our bright young people are unwilling to work as hard as did students eight or ten years ago. They believe that the attitudes of many of the faculty are unbalanced in terms of their views about what is important in life; they are often especially critical of those who devote much of their time to research.

We pride ourselves that our students have Medical College Admission Test scores in the 90th percentile and comparably high academic averages; yet after they reach medical school these same students are often disdainful of our traditional respect for and recognition of academic excellence. Being bright, they are able to "get by" academically, particularly at this point in time when grades are being de-emphasized. This de-emphasis reflects the fact that students do not want to be graded, they do not want to be ranked, and they do not want to take examinations. Many schools, rightly or wrongly, have gone along with their students in these areas. My concern is that in so doing we have created a situation in which our students are not utilizing their potential adequately.

The foregoing are rather negative comments, and in all fairness I want to make some positive ones as well. Most of us would agree that students coming into our medical schools today are sincerely interested in the health care of their fellow citizens and dedicated to its improvement. Their concern is especially directed toward the upgrading of health care for the disadvantaged groups in society.

This motivation is admirable, and one of our challenges is to try to help our students use it constructively. But whereas we have many great gaps in our health care system in the United States and agree that it is certainly far from satisfactory, it is difficult to see how quality health care is going to be administered by physicians who do not have an adequate concept of the relationship of science to medicine. The poor need better physicians not poorer ones. Some of our students seem unable to comprehend that one can understand the science of medicine and still be a good physician, interested in his fellow man in the broadest sense.

Let me cite an extreme example. In February 1968 at the annual Congress on Medical Education, a meeting of the medical school deans was disrupted by a group that was predominantly made up of medical students. (It is worth noting in passing that a number of the students who were leading the demonstration came from what are generally considered to be the leading medical schools in the United States.) One of them stood up and said, "We spend too much time educating people for medicine in this country. You can take somebody off the street and make him a good doctor in six months."

That is obviously not a view that most of us would accept, but the fact that a student from a first-class medical school would express it is alarming. It suggests that in their zeal to improve medical care some of our students have lost sight of what medical education is all about.

To some extent we medical educators are responsible for this development, and as usual we are responding after the crisis has occurred. But in a number of important ways we are responding; as already noted, we are changing our curricula in order to make them more meaningful to students and to avoid some of the unnecessary repetition that has existed.

Be that as it may, many students want everything to happen right now. Recently a leader in the Student Health Organization, an activist group, issued a statement saying that medical schools in the United States were so bad that there was no solution except to destroy them. There was no suggestion as to what he would replace them with. I doubt that this view is generally held, but it is disturbing even if held by only a few.

A number of factors contribute to the students' concern about medicine, of course. They are critical of the average practicing physician whom they perceive as being primarily interested in making money so as to live the "good life"; in their eyes his sense of values is badly distorted. Such a view is unfair to the many dedicated physicians who work hard and serve well. Nonetheless, the students believe that the average physician has too little concern for his fellow citizens.

To at least some extent, this perception reflects the fact that the American Medical Association, the organizational spokesman for a large segment of the profession, has not been, to understate it, the most progressive organization in the country. In fact, the A.M.A. has often opposed social change, especially in the medical area. Inevitably, therefore, the students attribute the A.M.A.'s attitudes to physicians in general.

At the same time, many students are also critical of full-time faculty members, whom they perceive as primarily interested in research and inadequately dedicated to teaching. To some degree there is a foundation for this accusation; our medical schools are heavily dependent on federal government financing, which is given almost entirely for the support of research, and faculty members do what they are paid to do.

Further, in most schools promotion to higher academic rank usually reflects research accomplishments. Medical school financing has been unbalanced and we have had inadequate funds for support of educational programs *per se*. The students see faculty members whom they consider to be effective teachers and clinicians passed over for promotion, while others, who may have done excellent research but who may not be interested or effective in teaching, are elevated. The students' concern about such matters is laudable. The problem we face is how to make the changes that are long overdue and to indicate to our students that we can react to constructive recommendations and correct injustices.

Students are particularly disturbed about many aspects of society as it exists in the United States today. Most of you are familiar with the kinds of problems we are facing. Our major cities are in crisis; they are overcrowded and mass transportation is grossly inadequate. The living situation for many urban dwellers is grossly unsatisfactory, and tension is accentuated in most of our large cities by the racial problems that have come to a head over the past decade or so.

Students as a group are critical of our foreign policy and particularly resent our involvement in Vietnam; this is a pervasive force in their over-all attitude. Many of us share this feeling, but students react more strongly. Further, our draft policy, which places a heavy burden on young males, is an added source of disillusionment and protest.

As with students elsewhere in the world, our students are concerned about the governance of the university. The procedure for policy-making in the university is grossly unsatisfactory from their point of view. I consider their concern reasonable and in large measure constructive, but they sometimes want to change the existing order in a way that is impractical.

As a group they are concerned about authority in all areas of life. Many are unhappy about their parents' values and ways of life, and there are times when we think that their unhappiness about their parents is being taken out on the university.

Obviously there is a spectrum of students. Some still go about their business as though life had not changed at all. But experience has shown that it does not take many activists to make a large issue out of one or another discontent, and there are some who work at this process diligently.

It has been observed by a number of medical educators in the United States that in the last year or so activism has been particularly common in the first and second-year classes; by and large, students who are near the end of medical school tend to be less activist. With students now coming into medical school who have been activists in college, it is likely that we will see more student unrest. To some degree, the locus of the medical school, that is, whether it is on or off the university campus, is important; when it is on the campus, the activism that involves the rest of the university usually spreads to the medical school.

The spirit of activism is now affecting our interns and residents, most of whom obviously graduated from medical school before activism became so much a part of the scene. For example, recently our hospital director was confronted by the interns and residents who demanded a $3,000 annual salary rise retroactive to July 1. This experience was a first, at least for us.

Some faculty members, particularly junior ones, are also dissatisfied with the hierarchical structure of the university. In my view, one of the major strengths of the student movement is faculty discontent. During Harvard's student uprising in the spring of 1969, the faculty was split right down the middle in terms of its view of the student position. When this happens, the administration, toward which much of the activity is ostensibly directed, is in a situation that is almost impossible to deal with effectively.

Many people have pointed out that the students' real target is the faculty and that the administration is merely a convenient whipping-boy. The complexity of the situation is great, notwithstanding the fact that the motive force is provided by a small group. Given a sensitive issue, they succeed in mobilizing large numbers of students on their side, and they then constitute a grave threat to the universities. I think at least some of the destructive elements really do want to destroy the institutions.

The participation of nonstudent activists is more of a force in the general university than it is in the medical school. The most notable example of this problem has been the Berkeley campus of the University of California, which for several years has had a nonstudent community on its periphery. In the past four or five years this group has grown and now includes hippies, a large drug culture, and a significant component of self-styled revolutionaries. The Berkeley situation seems at times beyond control, and the pressures on the university administration are enormous.

In many universities, especially those in large cities, there is a potential nonstudent group. Recently nonstudents have added to campus problems on an increasing scale in many locales, although interestingly enough, nonstudents were apparently not a factor at Columbia University when the unrest broke out there in 1968.

When student activists find that things are going against them they often issue an invitation to sympathizers from other areas to come in. In one of our uprisings at Stanford, a nonstudent, active in campus disturbances in the San Francisco area, urged the activists to "send out the word and we will be there in numbers."

In most of our schools students have been able to meet with deans and faculty at will, either alone or in small groups. But the concept of "participatory democracy" provides a new source of frustration because it is incompatible with any kind of representation. Thus we found that when students were appointed to the curriculum committee, others came to tell us that the representatives chosen could not speak for them.

We have to look at the situation realistically. If two students are added to a committee, some will want four. If the students are not in the majority, they will ask for enough additions to constitute a majority. In the last analysis, the advocates of participating democracy want every issue dealt with in a mass meeting where everyone can speak. I have not learned how to operate an institution on that basis.

Over the last few years increasing activism has been more prominent in a relatively small number of medical schools on the East and West coasts and uncommon in the southern part of the United States. Every now and then one of my colleagues will return from giving a lecture at a southern university and say, "You ought to go down there. You will find it very peaceful. The students still call you 'Sir' and behave themselves." But I venture to say that the kinds of changes we are seeing in our schools on the coasts will spread rapidly, and there is no question that they will affect all schools eventually.

In summary, as one who has been involved in medical education for twenty years, I would say that today's medical students have a great potential and motivation to make a meaningful contribution to society. On the other hand, they are so caught up in the problems of the times and in many instances seem to be so unable to direct their energies constructively toward the design of workable solutions that the situation is one of constant tension. Those of us who sit in administrative offices often wonder when the next explosion will occur.

Most of us who are responsible for the administration of American medical schools have great concern about what may happen in the next few years. It is entirely possible that the enterprise will be severely crippled unless we can persuade our students to be a little less impatient in their search for change. In the meantime, our job is to try to keep some balance. It is an interesting time but it is not a very happy one.

Germany

DR. SCHAEFER: The situation in Germany is almost exactly the same as it is in the United States.

I have been concerned with trying to figure out the reasons for the students' attitudes. I started by considering the students' psychology with the thought that perhaps I could learn something from a study of their personal histories. This led me to the following observations.

First, do a considerable number of revolutionary-minded students come from families that are in some degree disturbed? Recent studies of human psychology show that the very first years in a child's training have a decisive influence on his later social behavior. Some of the behavioral patterns of these student activists may, therefore, be explained on the basis of deviations in their early training and education.

My experience is that the most active revolutionary students in Heidelberg—and I have also observed this in Berlin—come from families with high social status; for example, they are the sons of professors and affluent industrialists. Some of the students have been in serious trouble at home.

This, of course, is an oversimplification and in my opinion does not explain the revolutionary movements at the universities; nor does it account for the fact that very similar disturbances in behavior are found in such different countries as the United States, Italy, France, and Spain, where the historical and economic backgrounds are so widely disparate.

It is obvious then that the reasons for this anomaly are not to be based on the social standards or recent histories of the respective countries, nor on the general psychological background of each country.

Yugoslavia

DR. DOGAN: Last year we had some trouble with our students who put forth some demands which we discussed with them. On the surface they are quiet at present, and we are trying to bring some order into the situation.

Our greatest problem is not with medical students but with students of sociology, philosophy, political science, and so forth. I believe this is true in many other countries also. Our medical students were less involved in last year's unrest, although the older students made specific demands, such as that they be given the title of M.D. They asked for more participation in the operation of the medical schools, because they felt they were being treated as children. They were very much concerned about their future after graduation.

I am not sure that the unrest has the same roots everywhere in the world. When I studied medicine in Yugoslavia, before World War II, the unrest was much worse than it is today, for it involved armed battles on the campuses. At that time it was caused primarily by political factors; today its roots are only partly political.

We have not made a thorough study of the psychological backgrounds of the students, and I think this is relevant only to a limited degree. The fact that only a minority of the students give us trouble is not as important as the fact that they have the sympathy of the larger group. In all revolutionary movements it is the more discontented individuals who initiate the action, and this is true in the case of the students. The more disturbed students are the most active, but as a minority they could not accomplish so much unless they had the support of the many others.

It is interesting that this general youth movement started in countries that have relatively high standards of living, especially the capitalistic countries. The students are asking for certain social changes, perhaps under the influence of some modern philosophers such as Marcuse, who visited Yugoslavia recently. Many of the changes that students are asking for in Germany, for example, have already been made in Yugoslavia, and yet our students still feel dissatisfied. Some of our students are obviously extremely left wing in their philosophy, but they cannot express their views openly in Yugoslavia because extreme leftist movements and anarchism are not tolerated.

My impression is that this is a changing generation and that the gap between the generations at this time is greater than was true formerly. I think it has become wider for various reasons and that there is a biological element involved.

In Europe we have had two wars in the last fifty years, and there has been unrest for twenty years following each war. I have talked to many students, some of whom belong to affluent families, and to a large degree they express disappointment with both their parents and their teachers.

POLAND

DR. JANUSZEWICZ: We have not had any trouble with medical students in Poland, but there was unrest in the universities a few years ago, led by students of sociology and philosophy.

Two years ago pedagogical councils were formed to study the organization of each year of medical studies and there is student representation on each of these councils.

As a group I think medical students in Poland are dedicated and enthusiastic and much better prepared now than at any previous time.

I am in charge of the pedagogical council in the third year of medical school and we spend much time discussing problems with the students. I think it is a good idea to have a free exchange of opinions and to hold these discussions as often as possible.

ITALY

DR. PAOLETTI: I do not think the student unrest in Italy and elsewhere should be considered as an independent phenomenon. In Italy the student unrest reflects changing patterns of student attitudes. Our medical students come from a small percentage of the population—the not more than 10 per cent that constitute the upper class. In this our students correlate fairly well with those at Stanford University.

These are the students who are more likely to induce unrest in our universities, but they have been successful in only one or two places, most notably in Rome and primarily for local reasons. Rome, with a total student enrollment of 90,000, is one of the largest universities in the world, next to Mexico City and Buenos Aires. The current medical school enrollment at Rome is 10,000, of whom 1,800 are freshmen.

The unrest has been very limited at the smaller universities, such as Milan with an enrollment of only 20,000 students. This may be due to the old-fashioned structure of our universities, where neither students nor younger faculty have any representation on the councils. The old-fashioned universities have proved to be extremely solid and unreactive, however, and I do not feel that this can go on indefinitely.

CHILE

DR. VIEL: The famous University of Cordoba revolution of 1917 was the first expression of student unrest in Latin America. It was a curious revolution that can now be analyzed from a different point of view than it has been in the past.

I have talked with several people who were students when the revolt took place and who are now on the faculty of medicine at the university. Cordoba had rather unique professors at that time. For example, the professor of anatomy was a landowner who came to the university only occasionally, usually when there was no harvest to be brought in. The students became very angry about such conduct, so they revolted and appointed committees of students to control the professors and their methods of teaching.

As the students began to exercise control over the faculty, and as the universities improved, they began to use the faculty seats they had taken over to fight for political power. Prior to World War II all Latin American student revolutions were politically motivated; they were devices to fight the government—to depose one president and put another one in his place. The students were not concerned with improving the organization of the universities or the curriculum.

In early 1968 our students went on strike against the old-fashioned system of medical education, but the feeling was even stronger among the assistants, the middle level in medical teaching, who were bitter about the fact that they were responsible for 80 per cent of the teaching and yet were not permitted to participate in faculty committees. The rebellion was not against society, although this was not the case in the university in general.

We are bitterly disappointed that after one and one-half years neither the assistants nor the students have come up with proposals to improve the curriculum or to reorganize the university.

The students believe that they are not being taught the kind of medicine that will be useful in the future, and they complain constantly that they are being prepared to become private practitioners to take care of the rich, when they will in fact be practicing in a different kind of society, one in which socialization will probably play a much more important role than it does now.

Although most of the universities are supported by the state, they are completely autonomous in making faculty appointments, and the people who hold these positions can be fired only by the university. But the students use the word "autonomous" in the same sense it was used by the Catholic Church in the Middle Ages—when a criminal took refuge in a church he was protected and the authorities could not touch him. The students want universities in Latin America to be sanctuaries that the police cannot enter.

This has been exaggerated in Latin America to the point where there are many examples of individuals who are not students living on the university campus and preparing bombs and other weapons in the laboratories. Some government authorities have found arsenals stored in the universities. The students, however, feel strongly that the university should be outside of the law; they do not want civil law to be applied on the campus.

About 2 per cent of the activists are nonstudents who live on the campus and are well protected because 90 per cent of the students fight the authorities when they attempt to get onto the campus.

Brazil

DR. SANTOS: A considerable amount of student unrest has occurred in Brazil under different guises for a good many years, but we have not learned to cope with it effectively. Now that it has spread to many other parts of the world I have been brought to the increasing realization that we know very little about the basic causes of the unrest.

In Brazil the reasons now being given for the student upheavals are entirely different than they were in the past. Ten years ago, for example, the students demonstrated very actively, because they maintained that teaching was slanted too much toward the humanistic aspects of medicine and not enough toward scientific and technological problems. Today they are demanding less science and technology, because they believe these are only preparing them to be the instruments of the ruling group.

We do not know the common denominators for the unrest; what applies in one part of the world certainly does not always apply in another. For example, I have seen demonstrations handled in a most sympathetic way and yet despite this they have become more violent. On the other hand, I have seen unrest handled brutally and, again, the situation worsened because the students became incensed over the brutality.

Students have always had initiative, and one would expect them to exercise it in demonstrations. Usually a particular episode will diminish after a certain period of time, somewhat like an epidemic that runs its course. We do not know what kind of antibody develops among the group—whether it arises naturally among the entire group or only in the leaders. We have attributed the end of an episode to different factors, while not really being able to pinpoint the true cause of it.

Many reasons that I do not consider relevant are being given for the student uprisings in Brazil. One is that the students are much better organized than heretofore—they are now organized on a nationwide rather than on a local scale. Another factor, which is the opposite of Professor Viel's experience, is that the most recent demonstrations have been much more politically oriented than in the past. Students used to protest more against local problems within the university, against a certain professor, or the format of the curriculum. Today they tend to support the university and to protest against the government and the organization of society.

There is something basic about the behavior of our youth that is not very well understood. One ingredient probably present in all parts of the world is that the students' concept of authority has changed. At one time they had respect for any kind of authority; there has been a change in this attitude.

It can be infuriating to deal with the student leaders or with large groups of students who are in revolt. One is often apt to lose control of oneself even though there may be some positive and constructive aspects to their demands. Until we know more about what we are dealing with I think the only solution is to remain calm and use one's personal judgment in any given situation.

Japan

DR. USHIBA: The Japanese system of medical education was imported approximately 100 years ago from Germany, where at that time medical science was the most advanced in the world. This fact has certainly influenced the quality of our medical students.

Following a period of national isolation, Japan was on her way to a period of civilization and enlightenment due to the introduction of modern foreign cultures. Some aspects of feudalism, such as the old family organization and the apprenticeship system, still existed, however, because of the long historical tradition in the nation. In such a feudalistic climate the research and chair systems advocated by world-famous scholars of the mid-nineteenth century, and the medical education method based on lectures, were introduced from Germany without meeting any resistance. What is surprising is that this system of education was maintained throughout the Meiji era until the end of World War II; some aspects of it remained even after the war, when so many changes took place all over the world.

When considering the characteristics of medical students in Japan today, we cannot ignore this history and national tradition. Before World War II most medical students came from the traditional family system. They wanted to follow their fathers' profession and were content to study under the apprenticeship system; some left their home towns with the dream of becoming great scholars or famous professors.

In about 1930 when I set my heart on a medical career I dreamed of serving humanity through medical research, but very few of my classmates showed a strong interest in the delivery of medical care, nor did they have a sincere desire to save lives.

Although today the social status of a physician is considerably lower, in those days it was as high as or even higher than that of other scholars. The students going into medicine were, therefore, the most elite of the elite because of the highly competitive entrance examination. But the ambition of this elite group was not to give the population better medical care, but to become world famous professors or scientists through great research discoveries. Unfortunately this tendency led to the present situation where some college professors still place more emphasis on medical research than on medical education.

Until quite recently medical students were inclined to be moderate and even conservative in their outlook, perhaps because formerly they came from families that could afford the heavy expenses of a medical education. Today the students' attitudes are changing rapidly, as can be observed in the case of the strife at Tokyo University which originated in the medical school. In fact, medical students in Japan are beginning to constitute the core of the radical group.

The reasons for the change in their thinking are not simple. One factor is that the rapid economic development after the war made it possible for people from various social groups to study medicine. Another is that with the general changes in society, medical students have gradually thrown off the feudalistic traditions and have become more interested in the social aspects of medicine. As sensitive young people they are beginning to feel dissatisfaction and repulsion over the conflicts existing in the present system of medical care and over the old-fashioned and imitative quality of our medical education system.

At this critical time many medical educators are still mainly interested in medical research and have been slow to appreciate the real meaning of medical education and the social aspects of medical care. All of these factors have accelerated the change in the medical students' outlook and have contributed to the unrest in the colleges.

In order to find the causes of our medical students' changing attitudes I surveyed the occupations of the fathers of Keio University medical students over the last ten years. The results (Table 1) show that no significant changes have occurred in occupations. The marked change that has taken place in the students suggests, therefore, that it does not originate in their families or social groups but in the general social climate.

An interesting point in Table 1, also, is that physician or medical practitioner fathers have constituted about 50 per cent of the total over the past ten years. Although this tendency is seen more often in private than in national schools it suggests that the traditional family system in Japan still exists, despite the changes in student attitudes.

Another factor concerns the difference between attitudes of medical

TABLE 1. CLASSIFICATION OF THE FAMILY PROFESSION OF MEDICAL STUDENTS IN THE TEN YEARS 1960–69 (SCHOOL OF MEDICINE, KEIO UNIVERSITY, 1969)

	Physician (general practitioner)	School educators	Public officials	Business	Shop holders, small business	Writers, lawyers, etc.	Farmers	Others	Unemployed	Total
Premedical										
First year	52 (40)	8	5	28	14	1	0	15	2	125
Second year	49 (44)	6	4	18	10	1	0	11	3	102
Medical Course										
First year	48 (43)	9	6	23	12	2	0	14	0	114
Second year	49 (49)	5	2	30	19	0	0	3	0	108
Third year	48 (43)	3	5	17	9	1	0	6	0	89
Fourth year	55 (52)	5	4	23	16	1	0	8	0	112
’69 graduates	39 (38)	1	4	15	19	1	0	5	0	84
’68 graduates	51 (47)	4	2	14	14	1	1	1	4	92
’67 graduates	35 (30)	3	3	19	16	1	1	5	3	86
’66 graduates	44 (35)	3	8	11	14	0	0	7	0	87
Total	470 (421)	47	43	198	143	9	2	75	12	999
Per cent	47.1	4.7	4.3	19.8	14.3	0.9	0.2	7.5	1.2	100

TABLE 2. MEDICAL SCHOOLS AND THEIR MATRICULATION (1969)

Medical schools		Fixed number of students in matriculation			
Status	Number	60	80	100	Total number of students per year
National	24	1	7	16	2,220
Prefectural and municipal	9	6	2	1	620
Private	13	2	4	7	1,140
Total	46	9	13	24	3,980

students in national schools and those in private schools, which seems peculiar to Japan. To explain this one must compare the tuition and other fees in both kinds of schools. There are at present 24 national medical schools, 9 public schools (prefectural or municipal), and 13 private schools. Total student enrollment as of 1969 is 2,200, 620, and 1,140 respectively (Table 2). The fees at the private schools are obviously high (Table 3). Furthermore, matriculation fees in private schools are remarkably high, as are the fees for facility expansion that must be paid upon admission.

Because of the large investment made in the education of private medical school students the unrest in the private schools tends to be mild compared with that in the other schools.

My final point concerns the changes in the learning capacity of medical students. This became apparent to some extent following the

TABLE 3. TUITION AND FEES IN MEDICAL SCHOOLS

	National schools	Prefectural or municipal schools	Private schools
Entrance exam fees	¥3,000 ($8.30)	¥3,000–7,000 ($8.30–19.40)	¥7,000–10,000 ($19.40–27.80)
Matriculation fees	¥4,000 ($11.10)	¥3,000–50,000 ($8.30–138)	¥100,000–350,000 ($277–972)
Annual tuition	¥12,000 ($33.30)	¥12,000–24,000 ($33.30-66.60)	¥150,000–250,000 ($416-694)
Laboratory fees (annual)	may be charged on actual cost basis	¥5,000–8,000 ($13.80–22.20)	¥5,000–50,000 ($13.80–138)
Extra fees for facility expansion		¥0–100,000 ($0–277)	¥200,000–350,000 ($555–972)

reformation of the curriculum after the war, but not to any striking degree. For example, in a couple of schools a new curriculum was adopted that greatly increased the amount of time for laboratory work and bedside teaching and decreased the number of didactic lecture hours. The aim of the program, however, which was that students should learn to think for themselves, was not always achieved. Japanese students in middle and high schools are accustomed to cramming knowledge under the old German-style curriculum that consists of many lectures and the memorizing of material for the entrance examinations. Such students cannot easily make the transition to independent study. In recent years, however, this conversion has been made gradually in the medical schools by placing emphasis on laboratory work and bedside teaching, although many schools are still giving cram courses of lectures without enough elective time. More elective time must eventually be allocated, and it is hoped that this will contribute to better study habits.

Denmark

DR. BRØCHNER-MORTENSEN: We have had some student unrest at the University of Copenhagen for as long as I can remember, but it did not become a serious problem until two or three years ago.

We have 20,000 students and between 2,000 and 3,000 teachers in the university. Probably only 2 per cent of the students are real activists, but until recently they were supported by about 50 per cent of the students.

The students want better facilities at the university, just as we all do, but they want them today or at the latest tomorrow. They want more emphasis on social developments and some of them want a completely new, undefined society with more personal involvement of the individual. They also want more participation in the various decision-making bodies of the university.

For several years we have had student representation on the curriculum committee and other medical faculty bodies. This spring the senate of the university decided that students should have one-third representation in all university bodies, including the budget committee, and one-half on the curriculum committee. Some students, however, do not approve of the representative system and feel that major decisions should be made at an open meeting and that every person present, student or teacher, should have one vote. To this the university has not agreed.

Last spring our medical students prevented us from holding faculty meetings on campus, so we had to meet in private houses; that crisis is over now. During the past few months the situation has changed: there are fewer and more peaceful demonstrations and the majority of the students are concentrating on their studies. Of course, we do not know if this situation will continue.

There is something positive about the student unrest. They are very socially involved young people. They are also very interested in the developing countries, although up to now few Danish physicians have gone to Africa or Asia. We expect that in the future a number of those who are now activists will take posts in such places as Indonesia and Africa.

Currently, the junior teachers are presenting much more of a problem than the students. They accept the representative system, but claim that all members of all bodies of the faculty should be elected under the one-man-one-vote system, regardless of whether they are full professors or junior research assistants. Theoretically this means that all seats, including the offices of dean, departmental chairmen, and laboratory chiefs, could be occupied by the most junior faculty members.

The younger teachers in the theoretical institutes of the medical school are now on strike, and almost all teaching was at a halt last week. They are asking for higher salaries, better research facilities, and fewer teaching obligations (the state, which pays their salaries, requires that they spend half-time teaching and the other half on research). They want better promotion policies and more full professorial chairs; at the same time, some of them want to abolish professorships.

The economic side of this fight is between the teachers' organization and the government, which pays the expenses of the university. We and the students are the victims. We really do not know what the outcome will be.

The Netherlands

DR. QUERIDO: During the past year the student unrest in Holland has been very well organized and politically guided. It has become so strong that it threatens to destroy the governance of the universities through such means as the demand for a one-man-one-vote system. That is the trend of the movement.

The Ministry of Education has notified all the state universities that it opposes the one-man-one-vote system and that in September or October of this year a preliminary law will be presented based on participation of all levels of the university—the senate, administrative and technical staff, and the students.

Nomination of academic personnel will be permitted only by faculty on an equal or higher level, thus assuring the quality of the vote. In the teaching section no more than 50 per cent of the students may be represented. With the expectation that not all students will participate, it is probable that a majority of senate and staff will be represented in the teaching section. That is the position being taken in the Dutch universities and it is being opposed by the students.

I think the best analysis of the situation appeared in James S. Ackerman's paper in the summer 1969 issue of *Daedalus* entitled "Two Styles: A Challenge to Higher Education," in which he states that there is the objective analysis style, which is the way the universities operate, and the engaged style, personal and existentialist, which is actually behind the whole student movement.

Our hope is that those students who sympathized with the engaged style have now recognized that they are being drawn into a political movement—that they are being used—and that in the coming months they will reject the activist group. If this happens another massive attack on the universities will be avoided.

Panel: The Curriculum

The Netherlands

DR. QUERIDO: I am offering a more or less futuristic view of medical education.

I am reminded of an expression used by an American friend who said, "It is more difficult to change a curriculum than to move a cemetery." As the dean of a new medical faculty in Rotterdam I started from scratch, and with my friend's pessimistic comment in mind I tried to be as innovative as possible. I could not be innovative in the real sense, however, because I was bogged down by the law applying to higher education that requires us to fulfill specific requirements.

The interest in changing the medical curriculum in the past decade has been worldwide and the reasons manifold. (The student unrest in this connection is of only very minor importance.) There are two directions in which people are moving in their attempt to reorganize the medical curriculum. One is based on the recognition that the curriculum during the student's years at medical school will play only a minor part in his professional life, because medical knowledge is changing very rapidly and that, therefore, it is important to educate the student to think independently. One sees very clearly this departure from a vocational type to a more fundamental type of training.

The other direction, which is probably more important to the developing countries, is that in order to raise the living standards of the community, preventive and social medicine are becoming essential elements in the curriculum and in the training of physicians. Both lines of development stress education more than professional skills.

There are many reasons why medical education is being scrutinized. The first is that medical sciences have come to maturity only in the last few decades. Professional training for medical care has existed for many centuries and has been supported by theories that have not been productive. In the middle of the nineteenth century Claude Bernard proposed that disease was an expression of a disorder of normal processes and suggested a methodology to study it. It was not until the twentieth century however that physicians had enough knowledge to offer a basis for intentionally influencing the abnormal course of disease.

On the one hand, biomedical technologies—radiology, electrocardiography, clinical chemistry, electroencephalography, etc.—were developed to trace abnormalities. On the other hand, biomedical technologies were developed for changing the abnormal processes by such means as anesthesia, surgery, intensive care, psychopharmacology, chemotherapy, transplantation, etc.

Most of these developments have taken place during the past thirty years. For the first time in the history of medicine, theories and basic knowledge have been developed that can be considered as a mature basis for the application of this knowledge to medicine, to the care of the sick, or to the prevention of sickness.

Another very important point is that the attitude toward medical care has changed from one of regarding it as a charity to one of regarding it as a human right as important as the provision of shelter and food. It has become a utility and, depending upon what kind of society one lives in, utilities such as transportation and communications are offered society either by large companies on a competitive basis or by the state.

The medical utility probably has the largest manpower requirement of any enterprise in the western countries. In the United States I believe it is now the second largest and eventually it will be the largest. It is a very unusual utility because it is performed to a large extent by human beings, while at the same time it has great investments in buildings and machinery.

It is clear that what can be offered to society as a utility depends on the amount of money available per capita, which differs from country to country. It is crucial therefore to get the most value for the money available. This means that people in whom much has been invested should perform only those functions for which they have been educated, not simple tasks that could be done by other, less trained individuals.

This raises the question of whether from an organizational and management viewpoint the delivery of medical care operates efficiently. I would say it certainly does not. Until now we have given attention only to specialization in this enterprise, not to the stratification of training that can be applied to different levels of the health care system.

On the one hand we have the maturity of the biological sciences and on the other the changing public attitude that regards medical care as a right. If one looks at parallel developments in the hard sciences one comes to the conclusion that they have developed their delivery of knowledge and skills along different lines. After the industrial revolution an educational system was developed for supplying technology to the hard sciences. The hard sciences started out with faculties of sciences, then they developed technical universities, and finally they departed from the tertiary educational level by introducing technical schools at the secondary educational level. Thus they built a complete system for having technical facilities operating at different educational levels.

The medical curriculum has gone in a different direction. While the problem has existed for only the past twenty to thirty years, the pattern has been to add new knowledge to a curriculum that was originally an apprenticeship system.

Some universities are trying to break away from the congested curriculum that has come into existence. Most medical schools teach normal structure and function first and then the abnormal. At Rotterdam we have tried to have an intermingling, with the accent first on the normal, and then, with more emphasis, on the pathological. It is still sequential, however.

The need for more specialization at different levels of knowledge and skills made me consider whether we should maintain this sequential order or intentionally break it up in a different way, namely, teach a mixture of normal and abnormal until one educational level had been reached, followed by an extension of knowledge in both fields to a second level. This would enable us to use the first level as a general formation stage not only for medical students but for others also, and to develop specialization at the second level.

This system would achieve two goals. In the first place, level-one students could continue in classic and new fields of paramedical professional training. Second, if these students wanted to go into medicine at a later date they would have to add a new level of knowledge instead of starting from scratch. The delivery of medical care in the future will require new types of professions that will bridge the gap between the nurse and doctor. This will enable the delivery of care to be more efficiently organized.

This concept is supported in my opinion by developments we have seen in the physical sciences. The study of inanimate matter developed after the industrial revolution, with the introduction of technology.

Since the study of the organization of living systems has advanced rapidly only in the past two decades, this fundamental branch of the sciences will now be followed by development of its own technology. Technology applied to biology has already developed to some extent in the agricultural and veterinary sciences, and will be applied to human biology, which will give rise to human technical biology. The important point is that biology is not a hard science that studies only inanimate matter. Biology is the study of the organization of living systems. It has developed its own technology only in the past thirty years. Accordingly there is no reason for our educational system to follow the same trends as the hard sciences did in past centuries.

To my mind the first step to be taken is to do away with the term "medical school" and talk about "faculties of biomedical sciences" that can supply a first level of general education and a second level of specialization, just as the faculties of science do. Both these levels can then be followed by training in professional skills. Making the delivery of medical care more efficient through better stratification of skills and knowledge will be a contribution to the vast problem of meeting the costs of and demands for medical care in both developed and developing countries.

GHANA

DR. SAI: We are trying to give our students an education that will make it possible for them to keep on educating themselves. At the same time we are trying to give them training in a limited number of hours in a limited number of schools.

The point in medical education at which it becomes necessary to specify not only general objectives but tasks necessarily differs from country to country and from region to region. Our students, quite rightly, want to be as good as doctors in other countries. At the same time, they are being trained in centers completely unlike those in most other parts of the world because they will confront quite different situations when they graduate. Not only do our students want to be educated men but they want to acquire skills that within reasonable limits will be equivalent to the skills of physicians who have been trained to practice under different circumstances. This creates a serious problem for us.

Although medical education in Ghana began in 1924 it was not until 1964 that the medical school really began operations. Immediately after graduating the first class we decided that it was time to take another look at the curriculum. In doing so the following observations were made.

Our general objective is that a doctor should have both a scientific and a humanitarian attitude toward medicine and that he should visualize it in its widest sense as a community service. Immediately one comes face to face with a situation where the entire community is demanding services that the doctor is going to have to provide for $2 or at the most $3 per head per year.

The physician should appreciate the interrelationship of all aspects of health services in the broader context of community health care. He should recognize the limitations of his knowledge, ability, and available facilities, and should know when to seek further help from his professional colleagues. He should be able to supervise paramedical personnel and learn to use their abilities in a co-ordinated and efficient manner. He should also, when called upon, be prepared to train such personnel.

He should appreciate that the study of medicine does not end with the attainment of the medical degree and learn to accept the obligation to continue his self-education.

These then are the broad objectives.

On the question of teaching them, our educational system is probably more archaic than the British system because they exported it when they were still using it. All the terms are the same: we have the O level and the A level. But the teaching methods are not at all similar. If anything, we need more modern teaching methods than are used in the western world because we want to build so much on secondary school education and so much more rapidly.

One major problem with medical education in Ghana is that all the medical students have A levels. There is no question that they are the elite of our scientific society. Only about 50 per cent of children in Ghana attend school and less than 10 per cent of them go on to secondary school. Perhaps 20 per cent of that number get the chance to reach the A level and only about 50 per cent actually get the A level. So these represent the cream of our potential medical manpower. There is no reason why these students should not do as well if not better than most medical students, and they would except for the fact that their previous experience has not prepared them for the complexities of the medical education system.

By the time they finish secondary school the students have not yet been taught how to *learn*. One major issue with curriculum development at present, therefore, is how to make our students learn to learn.

We think we can do this by allowing them much more time in the curriculum to work by themselves. We have decided to move away from the old method whereby, after graduation, high school students were required to spend one year in the university with no medical courses except a little social science in the department of preventive medicine.

They will now take a six-year medical course. The first year will be based mainly on social sciences because the students have to take a compulsory course in the university in "African Studies" and to pass an examination on that subject. We feel that if we build into that first-year course some elementary statistics, anthropology, sociology, and psychology, and carry through to the point where they go on to the basic sciences, we will begin to have a fairly good approach.

We have compressed into one year the basic science course (anatomy, physiology, and biochemistry) that formerly took five terms. The students are not happy about this, but we tell them quite bluntly that we must make some time for them to study the anatomy of the community and community health.

We then have four full years of clinical and paraclinical sciences, as we call them, during which time several things happen. There are two three-month periods of block teaching. Instead of physicians and surgeons giving separate lectures, systems are taken in groups. This may not be unusual in many medical schools, but we are introducing it as a new approach.

One complaint in the past concerned the number of repetitions: students in a pediatrics course would be taught something about electrolyte metabolism and abnormalities and then hear the same material in the surgical course. We never knew whether the students were learning or whether they were being confused. Lectures on electrolytes will now be one series and apply to all departments.

We are hoping to include a six- to eight-week elective period but I do not know whether we will be able to carry through on this. Elective periods require individual supervision and the medical school is under-staffed.

We have tried to cut down considerably on pure clerkships and we hope thereby that students will have more time to learn to learn. In this direction the Department of Preventive Medicine has tried to contribute by various means, one of which is to have the students participate in community health projects at the end of their first year. The initial project was a survey of housing conditions carried out jointly with the university's Department of Sociology, which has a demographic institute.

The Institute of Statistics and the Department of Psychology helped to prepare a questionnaire which the students were taught how to use. At the conclusion of the project the questionnaire was analyzed by a computer, and a few of the results were used for teaching purposes.

The students feel that this project was very useful in that it exposed them to their own community—many of them had not known that conditions were as bad as they really are. It actually made them learn how to learn certain things. We feel that this is a good way for them to learn preventive medicine.

At the next level, various seminars are held and the students are given a subject to research. Groups of four or more students, guided by a teacher from either clinical medicine or pediatrics, search the literature and mount student seminars.

In the fourth year, students are assigned to pediatric patients and visit the children after they return home. We tell the students in advance all the things we think they should know, and after the experience they tell us what they have found out and how they think the situation should be handled.

These are some of the directions in which we are moving.

I have not spent much time on basic curriculum because as I stated earlier it is very much the same as the British system. Our major differences lie in trying to make sure our students put in enough time on pediatrics, because that is a primary concern in Ghana. We also see that they spend enough time on preventive medicine. While this may sound as though the students are acting at the clerkship level, we view our health service and health program development as major exercises in doing what we can to prevent illness by whatever means are available. In this we feel that the physician should take the leadership and that medical care, especially in the hospital, should be put in the correct perspective in terms of available funds.

The examinations are quite difficult because there is an obsession in Ghana to be accepted by our former "masters," the British. We have the external examination system which is broken down into four parts: the second M.D., pathology and microbiology, pediatrics and obstetrics, and the finals. We are thinking of eliminating at least one of the examinations and making the finals more comprehensive.

Another challenge we have thrown out is that we should not have a 3:3:2 kind of structure, with three years of human biology structured toward a university degree. The course should be polyvalent so that we will be able to include a group we lack very badly—the medical technologists. They are not coming in because a student of high caliber will go into medicine. At present if he is not good enough he does not go into any paramedical field and this is something we want to avoid.

The final three years of the medical course are followed by a two-year internship program. The internship lasts for two years because we think that is the minimum length of time necessary to give the doctor the skills he will require as a generalist in the rural areas. The first year consists of normal medicine and surgery; the second is structured to give community health care, including pediatrics, obstetrics, and some minor orthopedics.

Among our difficulties is the antiquated school system and the shortage of staff. The small staff is dedicated but does not have extensive experience in teaching, so they have had to learn as they went along. As a result they lack time for their own further development. I do not know how long we can operate our medical school under these conditions.

When there is a shortage of staff it is very difficult to evaluate students in a meaningful way. Apart from the examinations, we make an attempt at evaluation when the student spends a six- to eight-week rural health attachment period with us in his last nine months in medical school when he is virtually a graduate. They come in groups of four and five and work within the community and it is possible for the staff to really get to know them. This is one way of testing how each student works in the community.

Germany

DR. SCHAEFER: There have been no changes in the medical curriculum in Germany during the past two years. Some recommendations have been made by the *Wissenschaftsrat*, the official scientific council of the West German Government. A second approach to the reorganization of medical training has been made by the Ministry of Health, which is responsible for the governmental training schedule of physicians (what we call *Bestallungsordnung*).

The latter system divides medical training into five periods. The first year coincides with the British first year of premedical studies and includes biology, physics, and chemistry. This is followed by a one and one-half year period in which the students study physiology, biochemistry, and anatomy.

I think we still place too much emphasis on anatomy, giving it as much time as physiology and biochemistry combined. We have tried to revise the curriculum so that anatomy, physiology, and biochemistry receive equal time. In my opinion even that is too much, but of course anatomy is an eternal science. One of my anatomical friends put it this way: "Even if all hypotheses of physiology were proved to be wrong and had to be replaced by better ones, the kidney will still be lying in the same place God put it." That may be, but how often does a physician use his anatomical knowledge during his professional life?

The second period concludes with an examination in physiology, biochemistry, and anatomy. We are planning to introduce sociology and biomathematics into this period.

The third one-year period consists of the theory of disease—general pathology, physiology of pathological processes, physiology of disease, radiology, biomathematics, genetics, and pharmacology. There is some clinical training on a more or less theoretical level, including the influence on body processes.

The fourth and fifth years consist of teaching in pathology, all clinical subjects, and ecology (social, preventive, legal, and industrial medicine, and hygiene). The examinations at the end of the fifth year are divided into nonsurgical and surgical-medical subjects, neurology, psychiatry, psychosomatics, and ecology.

The curriculum concludes with the equivalent of a one-year clinical internship, mostly in internal medicine and surgery. At the end of this period there is an examination and the graduate is licensed as a general practitioner.

Panel: Postgraduate Training Programs

Great Britain

DR. SMART: Postgraduate education in Britain is currently in a transition phase. We are moving very much toward the sort of postgraduate training that exists in Denmark but at the moment the situation is a little chaotic.

Training for General Practice

At the end of the undergraduate period there is a compulsory one-year hospital internship, with six months each in medicine and surgery or another approved subject. The internship period is considered to be the rounding-off process to the undergraduate period.

As soon as a physician finishes his internship and is registered he may go straight into general practice with little extra training, which in fact some do. There are official arrangements for training assistantships in general practice, however, and the majority of graduates take this course before entering general practice as assistants or partners. Some medical centers have developed schemes of special training for general practice. At Newcastle, for example, we have recently established such a three-year training course that, generally speaking, involves a period in hospital, a period in general practice, and perhaps a return to another hospital position. Throughout the course, lectures and other forms of instruction are given on topics such as the organization of practice, social services, and so forth.

Such training programs have tended in the past to flounder for lack of suitable applicants, because when a person enters such a program he receives the same salary as he would in a hospital post, which is considerably less than he would earn were he to go straight into general practice. Over the three-year period of the training course he will probably lose a total of from £4,000 to £4,500. While he will be qualified to do a better professional job upon completion of his training, it does not benefit him financially in any way. Consequently, although these programs are rather successful from the purely professional point of view, because of the lack of applicants, they are training only very key people whom it is hoped will be the elite of the general practitioners in the future.

Senior Specialists (Consultants)

At present hospital training is not formalized. In practice, a physician cannot be a specialist unless he is employed in a National Health Service hospital. In order to get a senior specialist or, as we call it, consultant appointment in a health service hospital he must have an appropriate postgraduate diploma that is usually given by one of the royal colleges. In addition, he must have occupied a suitable series of hospital training posts in which he has performed satisfactorily. In general, the length of time involved is about the same as in Denmark; it takes seven or eight years and sometimes longer from the time a physician completes his internship until he is eligible for a post as senior specialist in the National Health Service.

The Shortage of Physicians

As far as general training is concerned, the drawback is the discrepancy between the training that goes with a post in a large central hospital and that received in some of the smaller peripheral hospitals. In the large hospital some sort of educational activity is constantly going on, whereas the more limited resources of the smaller hospitals make such activity much more difficult. Furthermore, with a small staff the load of routine work becomes very great so that trainees may be left with far too little time to study.

Consequently the central hospital posts are very much in demand, with the result that, because of our very severe shortage of doctors, the peripheral hospital posts are staffed largely by people from overseas. This situation has struck the national conscience and has been a primary factor in producing the changes in postgraduate education that are now beginning.

Specialist Registers

It seems probable that Parliament will empower the General Medical Council to keep specialist registers. If this happens the G.M.C. will exercise the same control over postgraduate education that it has had over undergraduate education for the last 100 years. The training will, of course, take place in approved hospital posts and general practices;

universities will be concerned with general theoretical instruction and the over-all organization of the training. Postgraduate professional qualifications will continue to be granted by the various royal colleges, as they are at present, and these qualifications will be registrable.

For the purposes of the National Health Service the country is divided into regions. For example, the Newcastle Region, with a population of about 3 million, covers an area of about 120 miles from north to south and about the same area from east to west. The Birmingham Region, with a population of about 5 million, covers a much smaller area. Several regions go into London in wedges.

Each region, except those around London which are slightly different, has a university with an affiliated medical school. Responsibility for the administration of postgraduate training throughout that region, both in hospital posts and in general practice, will be placed jointly in the hands of the local university and the regional hospital authority. Most already have a postgraduate dean and/or regional director of postgraduate education who supervise the regional activities.

The cost of postgraduate training will be borne by the health service, insofar as it is vocational and professional; insofar as it is academic, it will be borne by the universities.

How is this plan going to be implemented? The general idea is that after internship all physicians—general practitioner and hospital trainee alike—will be required or encouraged to take three years of general vocational training that will be specialized to some degree; in other words the training for the surgeon will be quite different from that of the man who wants to specialize in medicine, radiology, or psychiatry. There will be some common overlap, however, so that a person may switch from one field to another—from pediatrics to medicine, for example—without losing a significant amount of time.

In the Newcastle Region we have begun such training with some of the posts in internal medicine. A person will do one year of general internal medicine at a peripheral (not teaching) hospital some distance from Newcastle. In the second year he will rotate through neurology, cardiology, and some options—he may do psychiatry for three months and, if he wishes, some pediatrics, dermatology, and so forth. In the third year he will do internal medicine in a teaching hospital. At the end of the three-year course he will be eligible to qualify for the appropriate postgraduate diploma; for an internist this would mean membership in a royal college of physicians.

There are three such colleges and they have now merged and grant one membership. Membership does not state that a person is a trained specialist in, for example, internal medicine, but that he is considered to have had the appropriate basic training to be a specialist after he has had further recognized training. It is essential to have that diploma before going on to the four-year specialist training period. Having obtained membership, a man training in internal medicine may go on to the next stage, which entails four years of training during which he may either do more general internal medicine or study a specialty such as neurology. In my region one of the four years may be a sabbatical in which the person may do research either locally or elsewhere. At the end of that year he returns to the same post in order to complete his training. Even though his training is finished, however, he must wait until he gets an appointment in the health service before he can be called a specialist. It is the conferring of the appointment that makes him a specialist.

It has been proposed that when a physician has completed this training and acquired the requisite experience (which will be specified by the G.M.C. on the advice of the appropriate royal college) he would automatically be given a post in the health service. He would have a certain amount of individual responsibility, short of the full specialist-consultant stage for which he would still have to compete and which he would ultimately be given.

At present there is an unfortunate dislocation in the hospital structure in Britain. There are far too many junior relative to senior posts, and were it not for the fact that about 50 per cent of the former are filled by overseas graduates (most of whom subsequently return home), many hospitals might have to close down. On the other hand, if they were all staffed by our own graduates it would be impossible to give all of them senior posts when their training was over. The Department of Health has already introduced measures to increase the ratio of senior to junior hospital posts.

Continuing Education

One other aspect of postgraduate education that is developing satisfactorily is continuing education for all physicians. There has not been much concern about hospital specialists, because they are usually in an atmosphere that ensures continued learning. It is very much more difficult for the general practitioner. The postgraduate dean of the university is largely responsible for organizing this training in his region, and there are a variety of ways this can be done. The university centers may, for example, conduct courses of a week's duration or perhaps for a half-day each week for, say, six weeks, so that a practicing physician may come in for a few hours a day each week. It has been noticed, however, that with this sort of course only about 25 per cent of general practitioners are constant attenders.

The problem is how to keep in touch with them. The most successful way so far has been to open postgraduate teaching centers in reasonably large hospitals. The university appoints a clinical tutor to each of the hospital groups, and he is paid an honorarium that the university collects from the Department of Health. The tutor is responsible for organizing postgraduate training in his group, which consists of both hospital personnel and local general practitioners.

The centers tend to be run as clubs, each having a library, lecture theater, and reading rooms. They may hold a luncheon meeting at the same time each week and have a lecture followed by discussion, or perhaps a case demonstration and a lecture. It has been found that this kind of function attracts most local practitioners, who have to pause for lunch anyway, and it enables the local specialists and clinical tutors to keep in close touch with them.

There are national courses for all categories of physician. Those for hospital specialists are usually conducted at the postgraduate institutes or schools in London, Hammersmith, Edinburgh, or Glasgow. A provincial center will seldom mount a national course.

General practitioners are encouraged by financial inducements to attend these postgraduate activities, for they must attend a certain number of courses a year in order to retain what is known as seniority payment. This amounts to only about £200 a year, but if they fail to attend the courses—and they may choose those they wish to attend—they lose the award. This is a surprisingly effective incentive.

There is another scheme for specialist-trainees or even established specialists who may apply to enroll in a highly specialized course. At Newcastle, for example, we have an internationally known center for the treatment of muscle diseases, located in our Department of Neurology under Professor J. N. Walton, who is well-known for his work on muscular dystrophy. If a specialist or a trainee-neurologist wants to go there for four weeks of intensive training in that particular subject, the Department of Health will pay his expenses and all of the fees. Most of the centers conducting this type of course are in London, but a number of provincial centers also participate.

In many regions every doctor receives a *Postgraduate Bulletin* which announces all of the courses and postgraduate activities in a particular region during the following four months, so that they are kept abreast of what is going on. In our region, doctors receive a publication called the *Adverse Drug Reaction Bulletin.* A very able physician began this project and every two months he writes two or three pages about a group of drugs to which patients may have serious reactions and describes how to counteract them. These are a few examples of what is being done to help physicians keep in touch.

Overseas Graduates

The activities I have outlined will improve the training that overseas people receive by many orders of magnitude, because they will begin to be involved in a properly thought out and carefully constructed rotation. At present, when an overseas graduate applies for training it is rather a matter of chance as to what sort of a post he gets and whether it is really suitable for his training. In the future, foreign graduates will apply to enter a program, as they do in the United States for a residency program, and they will rotate for perhaps three years and receive proper training. If they obtain a membership in a royal college at the end of that time they may then be able to elect to go on for further training at a higher level.

Poland

DR. JANUSZEWICZ: Recognizing the necessity for physicians to receive postgraduate training, in 1952 the Ministry of Health established the Institute for Advancement and Specialization of Medical Staff, which in 1958 was renamed the Center for the Advancement of Medical Qualifications.

The center is responsible for the postgraduate training of physicians, stomatologists, pharmacists, and so forth. Its function is to plan and co-ordinate postgraduate scientific programs.

Subsequent stages of training include compulsory basic hospital duty of two years' duration, specialization training of from four to six years, and continuing education throughout the physician's active professional life.

The basic hospital training is needed to obtain a license to practice, and it prepares the physician for independent work by increasing his practical knowledge. The training is rotated to include six months each of medicine, surgery, pediatrics, and obstetrics and gynecology. In addition, he has night duty in the emergency ambulance service and spends some time in the public health service system.

Upon completion of his hospital training the physician goes on to the next step which is training for a specialization. Depending upon the discipline, first- and second-stage specialization may be obtained. Each stage requires two to three years of training, followed by a specialty board examination.

In 1967, of the approximately 43,000 physicians in Poland about 13,000 had first-stage specialization and about 13,000 had second-stage specialization.

Of the three stages of postgraduate training the center is primarily concerned with the third—professional competence—and it takes an active part in specialization by establishing, for example, fellowships in such specialities as psychiatry and anesthesiology. Its activities are conducted through its chairs and departments in co-operation with medical schools and research institutes throughout Poland.

According to the 1965–66 figures, of the total number of physicians and pharmacists undergoing postgraduate training at that time, 49 per cent were enrolled in the center and 51 per cent in other medical schools and research institutes.

The center trains the chiefs of wards of district hospitals, large city hospitals, and country hospitals, and directors of out-patient services. The training is free and if a physician must take it in another city, free living accommodations are provided. He receives his usual salary during the training period.

The teaching program is prepared by committees appointed by the center, and their membership includes heads of departments at the center, national specialists, representatives of the Ministry of Health, directors of research institutes, regional public health service officers, and outstanding specialists in clinical disciplines. Such membership ensures a high professional standard and a many-sided approach to all aspects of the training program in order to meet the urgent needs of the regional health services and the most important requirements of particular specialties. Trainees' suggestions are also taken into consideration in preparing the program.

In order to give it wide publicity among health service personnel, the teaching program is published annually in the postgraduate center's own periodical and in other Polish journals.

Variety is the characteristic of current postgraduate training. The center sponsors several types of courses, such as basic, perfecting, informing, and verifying. Other aspects include seminars, scientific conferences, lectures, and grand rounds of hospital wards given by directors of teaching departments. The courses have different scopes and aims and vary in duration from one day to three months.

The noncontinuous training is a convenient form of education intended for local physicians and commuters so that it will not interfere with their regular work. Every month the center holds one-day panel discussions to which it invites outstanding specialists as speakers. Course participants are required to attend these meetings.

A good deal of attention is being given to regional training and the center plans to work out suitable methods and forms of postgraduate training for all physicians. It is generally believed that because of varying regional conditions and needs, such training should be in various forms. The regional training courses will be conducted by local health service authorities in co-operation with medical schools and medical societies.

Pressure is being put on the training chiefs of hospital wards and outpatient services to prepare good teaching personnel for regional programs. For example, in the academic year 1965–66, 25 to 30 per cent of all hospital ward chiefs completed postgraduate training in such specialties as medicine, surgery, pediatrics, and gynecology. It is expected that these specialists will direct the regional training and disseminate widely their newly acquired knowledge.

Postgraduate education in Poland is going through a continuous state of evolution in regard to both content and form. One advantage of the present teaching program is that it is revised annually, thus allowing for the inclusion of the latest advances in medicine. This system also enables the program to consider the actual needs of the public health system.

The extent of postgraduate educational training is illustrated by the data from 1967 which show that about 400 courses were organized and that about 4,000 physicians were trained. Two thousand physicians received first-stage specialization and more than 1,000 received second-stage specialization.

East and West Africa

DR. SAI: Now that we are looking to the future, one of the problems of postgraduate education for countries such as Ghana is the question of status. (Most of them have become status seekers rather than postgraduate education seekers.)

East and West African countries must start to take steps to plan for the students in our increasing number of medical schools, because it is inconceivable that we should not provide postgraduate education. In order to ensure outside recognition there is no reason why we should not have an English-speaking West African postgraduate training scheme covering all the colleges—perhaps under the wing of the Association of African Medical Colleges, which is now in its developmental stages.

I envisage assistance from the United States and Britain being channeled into the association to be used for local or regional postgraduate education. Initially this might require an external examination system.

There is no question that the Department of Pediatrics at Ibadan is the best in West Africa, just as the one set up by Dr. Jean Senecal at Dakar is the best in the French-speaking areas. A physician who wants to be a pediatrician could do his initial training at either of these centers and then return to his own country to be examined.

If we can get our East African colleagues involved in this kind of planning, by arranging for postgraduates to receive their training in various centers, or by bringing in teachers and mounting courses in selected areas, it should be quite possible to have a reasonably competent postgraduate program for parts of Africa, at least.

I am urging that the interested international organizations start thinking of postgraduate education for developing countries along these lines, putting in their resources to help locally rather than having our students go abroad for training that does not prepare them for the tasks that need to be performed in their own countries.

ITALY

DR. PAOLETTI: Postgraduate education in Italy is probably much better organized than undergraduate education. It consists of two different periods: The first year after the medical degree is granted is a form of compulsory postgraduate training in which the new physician spends about four months each in surgery, medicine, and obstetrics and gynecology. He then sits for a state examination and if he passes he becomes a member of the Italian Medical Association.

At this point he may apply to enroll in a first-level school of specialization, as we call it, where a very limited number of openings are available each year, ranging from ten to twenty in the basic sciences, biochemistry, or pathology, to about fifty in surgery or internal medicine. The length of training varies from three years in the basic sciences to five years in surgery and internal medicine.

At the end of this period he may go on to a second-level school of specialization where the openings are also limited—there may be as few as three places in specialized areas of medicine.

Because the schools of specialization have fewer students than the medical schools their programs are more versatile and there is a good deal of co-operation between the schools.

Students in some of the basic sciences (and in some specialized clinical fields such as surgery and genetics) are sent on a routine basis to foreign countries for six to twelve months' further training, while a number of foreign postgraduate students are accepted at our schools.

Continuing education is not so satisfactory because it is largely carried on by the medical associations and the pharmaceutical companies. In Italy the latter have no patents to protect them so there is very stiff competition for the market. For this reason they are interested in organizing courses and lectures for practitioners as a direct way to introduce their products. The pharmaceutical companies also distribute scientific literature and medical textbooks. (I should mention that Italians use more drugs than any other people in the world.) About 15 to 20 per cent of the gross earnings of the pharmaceutical companies go into some kind of education for physicians. This is a very high percentage compared to the 2 or 3 per cent that goes into medical research. I believe this is the opposite of what happens in many other countries.

The standard of continuing education varies considerably, but sometimes it is at a very high level. The medical associations hold local courses and conferences, chiefly for practitioners. There are no special requirements for enrollment in these courses, which may run for periods of a few days to as long as a few weeks, and no examination is given at the end.

The most recent survey showed that about 40 to 50 per cent of physicians in Italy go to the meetings organized by the pharmaceutical companies or by the local medical associations. This attendance rate is very satisfactory in view of the fact that it is not compulsory. Some standard should be set, however, in order to find out how well the courses are received and how effective they are in disseminating the increasing amount of medical information.

Panel: The Governance of the Medical School

Introduction

CHAIRMAN BOWERS: One of the most challenging problems a medical school dean faces in the United States today is governance—where the power is. How does one bring a faculty of medicine together as a cohesive unit? How are decisions made? What can one look forward to in the future? The Macy Foundation is interested in these problems and is involved in a nationwide study of the governance of the academic medical center.

Governance varies in different parts of the world and the United States is perhaps the only country where a man enters the deanship as a career. Elsewhere most deans take it as a post that they fill for a stated period of time, during which they retain their faculty and departmental appointments and in due course return to them. The pattern differs considerably but the problems are the same in varying degrees in all parts of the world.

Another point we have touched on at this conference is the rise in power of medical students in governance, and the insistence of younger faculty members on participation in decision-making in the school.

We have, on the one hand, the erosion of the power of departmental chairmen; on the other hand, the chairman stands as a significant factor in governance.

I think it is appropriate that our final session be on the governance of the academic medical center.

United States

DR. LUCKEY: The typical United States medical school as a part of the university has run a somewhat different course than universities in general. It is important to recognize that American universities grew out of the old Anglo-Saxon tradition of learning for learning's sake, the Germanic tradition of research for research's sake, and the same sort of utilitarian approach characteristic of university systems all over the world—direct delivery of service to the community. In the United States this had its origins in about 1865 with the passage of the Land Grant College Act, the so-called Morrill Act, that established colleges of agriculture and other units of the university that were concerned with the development of certain enterprises of immediate practical importance to the community.

The medical schools evolved differently, beginning as trade schools. Following the Flexner Report of 1910 they did take on university characteristics and in fact outdid the universities in their dedication to learning for learning's sake and research for research's sake, splitting the service activities of the hospitals as separate enterprises.

That historical background is important to recognize as it relates to governance, for in the beginning it did not take a large central structure to administer the programs of a community of scholars primarily concerned with educating and teaching a group of students.

When research is self-generated, without the kind of high organization that occurs when large amounts of funds are available, it does not complicate the matter of central administration nor, for that matter, affect the co-ordination or communication between professors or between departments.

In the early days in the United States, as I am sure was the case in other parts of the world, the central administrative structure of the medical school was small, temporary, and unimportant. There was a faculty secretary who was called the "dean of the medical school," a part-time individual who taught in the medical school and at the same time carried out all the administrative responsibilities of the dean.

Most medical schools maintained this pattern of the part-time deanship until the development of the full-time faculty that probably had its really important beginning in the University of Chicago in 1925 and developed in other medical centers shortly thereafter.

The presence of faculty members who needed to have a central system to co-ordinate their efforts and a chairman to function in that role led to the heightened importance of the role of the dean of the medical school.

But the major development in the increase of the need for deans took place after World War II with the enormously expanding budgets of the medical schools—consisting primarily of funds for research purposes. Burgeoning faculties, doubling in size every two or three years, made it necessary to have some one person to represent the image of the institution to the agencies from which it was to request funds.

In some respects this was not a happy period, but it was one in which the dean's role became so time consuming that it was necessary to begin to appoint more full-time deans. In fact, even fifteen years ago very few of the then eighty or so institutions in the country did not have full-time deans.

The dean of the medical school was often selected because of his standing in the academic community as a teacher or scholar. Very often he was an individual with important research accomplishments, or who had reached a dry period in his research, who was able through persuasion, cajolery, and often simply passive obstruction to influence the course of events in the institution.

Some attempted to play activist roles, but there is an inverse relationship in the United States between activism on the part of a dean and his tenure. Without any question, the individuals who have had the longest tenure are those who have reflected the most conservative influences in the faculty. That is not a derogatory statement; it happens to be true.

During the period from 1946 to 1966 the center of power in the medical school was undoubtedly the department chairman. The medical school chairman was appointed along the traditional lines that started at the Johns Hopkins University, and there was no limit on his tenure. Initially, in each department there was a single professor who was chairman and *the* authority in that department.

In the councils that represented the governing group within the institution—faculty committee, executive committee, and so on—although the dean would act as chairman, the departmental chairmen without any question were the most influential figures. Such faculty committees, with the dean as chairman, usually served very much in the role of both the board of governors and council. The chairmen of basic science and clinical departments sat around a table representing a consortium of oligarchies each of which operated quite independently. It was very much like the Security Council of the United Nations—by simply passive obstruction one could veto any important move.

Furthermore, because of the fact that they were supported not so much by institutional funds as by funds obtained from outside agencies, these departments were largely autonomous. For example, in the department that I headed for ten years, which had an annual budget approaching $4 million, only 25 per cent of the salaries of some 400 full-time faculty members came from hard-core institutional funds of the hospital and the university; most of the funds were raised each year from outside sources. The National Institutes of Health represented the largest source, but private foundations were important also.

The governing body of the institution of which the medical school was a part rarely played much of a role in the important policy-making decisions of the medical school, often being concerned with other somewhat more immediate and pressing problems of the university in general.

The students had little voice in the academic executive committee, nor did the community except as it related to institutions with which the medical college was affiliated and on which it was quite dependent.

In the United States less than one-half of the medical schools, primarily the state schools, have what one might call a wholly-owned, associated university hospital. A few private schools, such as Vanderbilt, have hospitals that are a part of the corporate structure. The Johns Hopkins Hospital, for example, is not—it is a separate hospital that co-operates closely with the medical school.

For resources for clinical teaching and for clinical laboratories the medical schools had to become dependent on other institutions, such as municipal, state, veterans, and federal hospitals, and on an array of private institutions, usually nonprofit, voluntary hospitals.

Because of this situation the patient-care needs of a community were often expressed quite clearly and the medical school had the opportunity of exposure in this connection. I do not want to paint too depressing a picture, but the medical schools were not concerned primarily with the communities they served.

I agree with Dr. Glaser that there were both important advantages and disadvantages in the too rapid expansion of funding for new medical research. I believe it was done at a rate well above 15 per cent a year, and we went through a period when a great deal of mediocre research was supported. The faculty became spoiled to the extent that they could support almost any project they wished with funds from outside sources. Requests to the dean and to the central administrative structure of the university were not very important to them because they could obtain such funds from other sources. This tended to divert the loyalty of the faculty from the medical college and the university to outside agencies.

That was the situation that three years ago led to a conference at which the Macy Foundation attempted to identify problems in the governance of academic medical centers; the conference had representation from a whole congregation of institutions in addition to medical schools. The conference in turn led to a survey over the last three years that has attempted to identify these problems in a sample of several medical centers. We do not as yet know the final conclusions of the survey, but one can make some statements that relate to the topic of this panel.

First, there is no question that we have a problem in the governance of our medical schools, centering around the fact that the organization as it now exists is ineffectual in its central planning. A consortium of oligarchies with a short-tenure dean and a long-tenure department head cannot function effectively in long-range plans for the school.

Second, it is perfectly clear that enormous changes are taking place in the communities that our medical schools serve and that support the schools.

One of the most important themes that every person at this conference has expressed in a different way is that all of us are becoming much more concerned about responding to community needs than has been the case in the past. We have spent a great deal of time here talking about the task-oriented requirements of medical schools, and we are all interested in this. It seems to me therefore that our governance structure is going to have to be modified to meet this task-oriented approach to our mission. We would like to protect the best of what we have had in the past and superimpose those things that will give us this kind of task-oriented governance structure.

As I have listened, it seems to me that we are saying that the community of scholars that represents the university is going to have to recognize that the constituency involved in this whole matter is much larger than simply a group of professors sitting around a table. If we are going to become task-oriented we must recognize that we have to work out some kind of satisfactory rapprochement with the health services of the country in which we are working. Not only the professionals in the health services but individuals who are being served by the services are going to need to be involved in our governance structures.

This is not going to be a simple matter for the proprietary interests or governing boards in our respective countries. The proposal is sufficiently highly developed and defensive that it is going to be very difficult to sell, particularly to our private, nonprofit, voluntary institutions. It will be hard for them to accept the idea of health services and community representatives being involved in governance, but it is inevitable that this will happen.

Another theme I have heard is that, with the possible exception of one or two countries that have an adequate supply of physicians, all of us are concerned about the fact that regardless of the stage of development of health services we are not going to be able to provide for the health needs of our people by traditionally trained physicians alone. Every country seems to be working on this aspect of the problem.

This is not unrelated to governance because whenever we touch on this problem we are immediately involved in the question of whether or not our products are acceptable in the market place. I think the United States is going to be one of the hardest to deal with from this standpoint.

But perhaps the most important problem, which we have not talked about very much in this meeting, relates to the character of the academic medical centers. During the period of very rapid growth of faculty size, research funds, and total institutional budgets, there tended to be a large congregation of diverse institutions—varying in role from academic to direct patient service, and in corporate structure from governmental to private (and often religious)—that tried to cooperate in the absence of a central governance structure. Good will and faith were the only important common denominators and one's perspective about virtue varied, of course.

All kinds of problems have arisen as a result of this complex we call the academic medical center. How does one get this congregation of institutions to work effectively with other agencies within the community in the delivery of patient service, while at the same time protecting the traditional precious opportunity of the university to teach and to find new ways of doing so? To me this is a crucial problem and I will be very surprised if our governance commission study does not identify it as one of the central problems of governance. We have no answer for it at the present time.

One special problem in the United States that may not exist elsewhere is that with the growth of health profession schools—medicine, nursing, dentistry, allied health professions, and pharmacy—very often the dean, who is the first-line academic officer in the medical school, relates to the university hierarchy through a second and, in some rare instances, a third professional individual—a vice president or vice provost for health sciences. This has caused complications in trying to divide administrative responsibilities between these two individuals. In many institutions it has resulted in such chaos that one or the other of them has had to resign.

My final point relates to a situation that has existed for the last twenty-five years and that I think is changing rather rapidly: As funds from outside sources have become less available, faculty are now turning to the university institution and thinking more in terms of the cohesion of the institution. Certainly the dean's position is more highly respected in terms of his obtaining funds from endowment income, in the case of private schools, and from state legislative appropriations in the case of state schools.

I have the feeling that as there is an increase in institutional appropriations to health-care demonstration programs and research in the delivery of health services, it will be different than it has been in the past with project research support. In project research support there was a divisive influence; the kind of large block grants that will come for other purposes is apt to be a cohesive force.

Obviously communication between student groups all over the world is as good if not better than it is among us. Most of us would recognize the extent to which there has been acquiescence on some of these questions. Is there evidence that there is any kind of international student movement? (I am not referring to a political movement.) It is interesting to me that the pattern is taking such a common form in all parts of the world.

This group of conference participants is probably as tolerant of change and as cognizant of the difficulties that exist in the university structure and in some of our archaic patterns as any group in the world. What troubles me is that if the international university system is in danger of destruction we ought to treat it as some kind of international epidemic.

If an epidemic were threatening the world, as a community of nations we would probably call upon the World Health Organization. Communications being what they are today, if the epidemic goes too far in one area of the world this pattern is going to be taken up in other parts of the world. So if students now have 50 per cent representation on governing bodies in France, Spanish students are going to demand equal representation.

It seems to me that certain reasonable standards could be set down by international groups so that we would not wait until the students made a demand but agree to it, saying, at the same time, that we will not go beyond that point.

The current situation is reminiscent of the movement of certain organized groups in the United States, and elsewhere, where one union will get an increase in wages and so another union asks for the same raise; each one fights to see which can get the most benefits and eventually there is an inflationary spiral that ruins the economy of the country. I am troubled by this because we seem to be in a stepwise process of attrition.

CHILE

DR. VIEL: The University of Chile has a very traditional faculty. The Faculty of Medicine consists of the schools of medicine, public health, midwives, and technical laboratory assistants. All are under the direction of the dean and each has a director. In the past the dean was elected by the faculty and he in turn appointed the directors.

Extraordinary professors were required to write a thesis and sit for an examination after which they received the degree of professor and earned the right to teach. From this group the faculty elected a professor when a chair became vacant, and because of this method of selection most of the professors were rather old. Little by little the faculty became an aged group.

It has been said that a council of very old people is like a car without a motor. By the same token, since the revolution in 1968 that brought in a young group, we are finding out that a council of very young people is like a car without a brake.

That is the problem we are facing now. The old faculty has been deposed. The deans are now elected by a committee with 25 per cent student representation, 40 per cent junior assistants, and 35 per cent full professors.

At present we are seeing a kind of fever of reformation, so it is very difficult to describe where the power is. We have what the university calls a senate that is in the process of devising a new law that will be enacted in November 1970, so they have a year in which to draw it up.

In the meantime the old law is not being enforced, so we are functioning on an individual basis. Each department is doing its best but there is no central organization. The only central power that exists is that of the treasurer who is distributing funds according to the old law.

It seems to me that some of the complaints of the students are quite reasonable. They recognize that in Chile today our society wants medical care delivered by specialists. The students are therefore seeking specialization early in their training; while still in medical school they are planning to become psychiatrists, surgeons, internists, ophthalmologists, and so on.

Some professors in the medical schools are encouraging early specialization by telling the students that medicine is a very difficult subject whose scope is so wide that no human being can hope to retain the entire body of medical knowledge; others are encouraging the students to become general practitioners. This division in the attitude of the professors is one of the reasons we are in trouble.

The solution the students are requesting is not a bad one. They are asking for the integration of clinical and basic sciences and an early division in medical studies in order that they may spend 30 per cent of their time in medical school studying some general field such as medicine, or a specialty such as obstetrics and gynecology, or pediatrics. In this way the general practitioner in the community would be replaced by a team of at least three individuals—an obstetrician-gynecologist, a pediatrician, and an internist.

In former times the deanship of the medical school was a technical, social, and diplomatic position. Now it has become a technical position only, and that is why we are requesting that the deanship be a full-time career. But I wonder who will accept that job. The man who does will have to give up all of his other interests and, at the rate things are going, it is very possible that he will be out of the university in a few years. We have not found anyone in our university who is willing to sacrifice himself in that way.

West Germany

DR. SCHAEFER: The situation varies considerably in Germany depending upon whether or not a university has adopted a new constitution. Heidelberg has, and under it representation on all decision-making bodies of the university consists of 25 per cent each of lifetime professors, nonlifetime professors, assistant professors, and students.

The students do not have the right to participate in the appointment of faculty members—we still maintain the principle that no person may vote on an appointment at a level he has not yet reached.

Up to the time we adopted the new constitution, the University of Heidelberg had not undergone any changes for almost a century. Its new structure will be completely different, more or less similar to Italian and French universities.

Poland

DR. JANUSZEWICZ: The Academy of Medicine in Poland consists of a Faculty of Medicine, Faculty of Pharmacy, and Division of Stomatology. The academy is completely separate from the universities and is under the authority of the Ministry of Health.

In the Academy of Medicine at Warsaw we have sixty chairs. The rector is appointed by the ministry and there are three vice rectors, a dean, and three vice deans.

We have a senate and a faculty council whose membership consists of the extraordinary and ordinary professors and doctors, chiefs of services, and assistant professors. All heads of departments are elected by the council.

In the coming months I think the structure of the academies of medicine will be completely changed. There is a tendency to abolish the chairs and to combine a few chairs into one institute. The purpose is to concentrate manpower and the training and research facilities in one large unit.

YUGOSLAVIA

DR. DOGAN: Over the years we have grown accustomed to some of the problems of governance and they do not seem to be as serious as when they first arose.

During the period just after World War II, when many social changes were taking place in our country, almost every aspect of life was strongly state controlled. We are steadily moving toward decentralization which at present is in an advanced state.

When the universities became decentralized the faculty was given a great deal of power but the president and/or rector represented the university. Since then the universities have drawn up some general rules concerning the standardization of teaching, election of faculty, and so on.

The process of decentralization eventually reached the medical schools which had been severely criticized because they were closed societies—strongholds resembling medieval castles with armies inside.

Seven years ago the hospitals were separated from the medical schools. Up to that time they had been integrated with the schools both financially and administratively. In separating them the idea was that the hospitals should be to a greater extent involved in community health services. It was also felt that it is not good for students to see a select group of patients who are not really representative of the normal patient population.

Since then the hospital staff has led a double life. As members of the faculty they are responsible to the dean of the medical school, and as members of the hospital staff they are responsible to the director of the hospital. They derive their income equally from the medical school and the hospital. The department chairmen are important persons at the school and at the hospital but have no special position in the faculty. There is no board of chairmen, they are simply members of the general faculty body.

At Zagreb I preside over a monthly faculty meeting. We have committees that act as advisory bodies. The students are members of these committees and when they attend the meetings they are co-operative. Neither the students nor the younger staff assistants have membership on the faculty board, but we do invite them to meetings if decisions are to be made that are important to them.

All the universities in Yugoslavia had trouble with students last year. I met with students at Zagreb for three days, almost twenty-four hours a day. They are quiet now and do not seem to have the strength to start again. Last year they did not know exactly what they wanted, but they have now organized and are putting forth their demands very clearly.

The current president of the university communicates very well with the students. His idea is to try to strengthen the university by integrating the departments while leaving the schools as autonomous units. The students agree with this scheme.

The students are asking for one-third participation in the university council, which is the main governing body of the university. But according to the rules we are now drawing up, we will have another body called a pedagogic-scientific board—something like a university senate—on which there will be faculty representation.

The students have asked for little or no participation on this board but they have asked to have a student vice rector at the university. We have no good reason not to consider this request, because we do not think the students are a dangerous element in the university. If they are co-operative we think we can deal with them.

INTERNATIONAL MACY CONFERENCE

"World Trends in Medical Education: Faculty, Students, Curriculum"

Villa Serbelloni, Bellagio, Lake Como, Italy
September 21–27, 1969

PARTICIPANTS

Daniel Bargeton, M.D.
Assistant Dean and Head
Department of Physiology
Université de Paris
Faculté de Médecine
45, Rue des Saint-Peres
Paris 6e, France

K. Brøchner-Mortensen, M.D.
Professor of Internal Medicine
University of Copenhagen
Faculty of Medicine
Blegdamsvej 9
2100 Copenhagen Ø, Denmark

Lowell T. Coggeshall, M.D.
R.R. #3
Foley, Alabama 36535, U.S.A.

José Cuyegkeng, M.D.
Executive Director
Association of Philippine Medical Colleges
547 Herran Street
Manila, The Philippines

Sergije Dogan, M.D.
Dean
University of Zagreb
Faculty of Medicine
Trg Marsala Tita 14
Zagreb, Yugoslavia

Antonio Gallego, M.D.
Professor and Chairman
Department of Physiology and Biochemistry
Universidad de Madrid
Facultad de Medicina
Madrid 2, Spain

Robert J. Glaser, M.D.
Dean
Stanford University
School of Medicine
Stanford, California 94305, U.S.A.

Wlodzimierz Januszewicz, M.D.
Director
Second Department of Medicine
Academy of Medicine in Warsaw
Ul. Nowogrodzka 59
Warsaw, Poland

E. Hugh Luckey, M.D.
President
The New York Hospital—Cornell Medical Center
525 East 68th Street
New York, New York 10021

J. S. W. Lutwama, L.M.S., M.B., Ch.B., M.R.C.P. (Dublin)
Dean
Makerere University College
Faculty of Medicine
P.O. Box 7072
Kampala, Uganda

Rodolfo Paoletti, M.D.
Professor of Pharmacology
Institute of Pharmacology and Therapy
University of Milan
Via Vanvitelli, 32
20129 Milan, Italy

Andries Querido, M.D.
Dean
University of Rotterdam
Faculty of Medicine
Rotterdam 2, The Netherlands

Sjahriar Rasad, M.D.
Dean
University of Indonesia
Faculty of Medicine
Salemba 6
Djakarta, Indonesia

Frederick T. Sai, M.B., B.S., B.Sc., F.R.C.P. (Edin.)
Professor and Head
Department of Preventive and Social Medicine
University of Ghana
Ghana Medical School
P.O. Box 4236
Accra, Ghana

Roberto F. Santos, M.D.
Rector
Universidade Federal de Bahia
Rua Augusto Viana
Salvador, Bahia, Brazil

Hans Schaefer, M.D.
Professor and Chairman
Department of Physiology
Universitat Heidelberg
Akademiestr. 3
6900 Heidelberg 1, Germany

Virgil C. Scott, M.D.
Associate Director
Medical and Natural Sciences
The Rockefeller Foundation
111 West 50th Street
New York, New York 10020, U.S.A.

George A. Smart, M.D., F.R.C.P.
Professor of Medicine and Dean
The University of Newcastle Upon Tyne
The Medical School
Newcastle Upon Tyne NE1, 7RU, England

* Daizo Ushiba, M.D., Med.Sc.D.
Dean
Keio University
School of Medicine
Tokyo, Japan

Benjamin Viel, V., M.D., D.P.H.
Professor of Hygiene and Social and Preventive Medicine
Universidad de Chile
Escuela de Medicina
Andes 4242, Casilla 12034
Santiago, Chile

* Prem N. Wahi, M.D., F.R.C.P. (Lond.)
Director General
Indian Council of Medical Research
Ansari Nagar, New Delhi 16, India

John Z. Bowers, M.D.
President, Josiah Macy, Jr. Foundation
277 Park Avenue
New York, New York 10017, U.S.A.

* Neither Dr. Ushiba nor Dr. Wahi were able to attend the conference but the papers they prepared are included in this volume.

INDEX